ACHIEVE MAXIMUM HEALTH

COLON FLORA

The Missing Link
in Immunity, Health & Longevity

DAVID WEBSTER

LIBRARY OF CONGRESS CATALOG CARD NUMBER: 95-79062

Webster, David, 1930-

    Achieve Maximum Health

    Colon Flora: The Missing Link in Immunity, Health & Longevity

ISBN 0-9647537-1-5

Medical Editor: Pamela Edmunds

Cover Design and Art: David Evans

Book Design: Beth Hagman

Final Review Editors: Beth Hagman and Heidi Clevenger

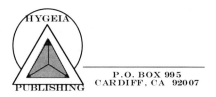

P.O. BOX 995
CARDIFF, CA 92007

The information contained in this book is not a prescription, makes no claims to cure any condition or disease and does not take the place of consultation with a physician. The information in this book is offered for educational purposes only. The author is a health research author and originator of the Webster Implant Technique. He is not a medical doctor and does not diagnose, prescribe, consult or correspond with individuals with regard to their health. If you are ill, consult your physician.

Permissions

Book Illustrations:

1. The following illustrations were used and modified with permission from Williams & Wilkins Electronic Media, from their *Medical Illustration Library, General Anatomy Collection II*. Macintosh version, Baltimore, MD. © 1994 Illustrations GA2-3002, GA2-2015, GA2-1031, GA2-5005. Figure 4: pH of Digestive Tract in Health, Figure 5: Portal Vein System, Figure 6: Unhealthy Colon Function, Figure 7: Healthy Colon Function, Figure 8: Lactobacteria pH Relative to Digestive pH

2. Background in cartoon courtesy of T/Maker Company, Mountain View, CA. From their Click Art® Images Collection "Skyline" image. ©1984 to 1993

Dedicated to my wife, Suzanne Eve Sky,
and to our angel

Table of Contents

Preface

Part I   The Foundation

Part 2   The Fall

Part 3   The Journey

Part 4 The Foundation Restored

Appendices & Endnotes

Pictures, Tables & Charts

Acknowledgments

My heartfelt gratitude goes to my medical editor, Pamela Edmunds, whose treatment of the rough drafts made the content understandable.

Richard Renn, D.O. Without his help, this work would not have been realized today.

Francis Gibson, D.C., who inspired me.

To Mr. Fritz, who handed me Dr. Empringham's manuscript, which was the driving force behind my work over the past 20 years.

To Mr. Max, our springer spaniel, who helped with his great spirit for 11 years.

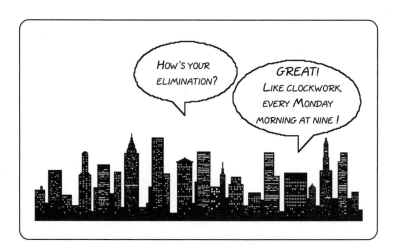

Preface
An Unexpected Avenue:
The Toxic Colon

In late 1974, at the age of 44, I experienced a surprising turn in my usually excellent health. One morning, I could not get out of bed; I was immobilized by excruciating pain in my left hip. For the next three days, I lay on my back, hoping the pain would subside.

Four days later, still in pain, I went to see a medical doctor. Although he subjected me to an extensive examination, he could not find the cause of my problem. He advised me to take Tylenol® and to learn to live with my discomfort.

Next, I sought the help of a chiropractor. I was again subjected to a rigorous evaluation process. Even thorough x-rays of my spine and hip gave no clue as to what was causing the shooting pain in my left leg. In despair, I returned home to read my health books, struggling to find the answer on my own.

My research led me to explore an unexpected avenue: the toxic colon. I found a chiropractor who offered colon hygiene procedures and made an appointment to see her that day. When I arrived at her office, I was still in great pain. During the colonic session, she assessed that my condition was an attack of sciatica, resulting from toxicity and an impaction in my colon. She explained that the largest nerve in the body, the sciatic nerve, can become inflamed due to an accumulation of toxic metabolic by-products from the colon. Such inflammation results in shooting pain in either the low back or the inside of the leg.

She went on to explain that an estimated 60% to 90% of the population experience this malady at some point in their lives. In the United States alone, the approximate annual cost to patients for treating sciatic nerve inflammation is 16 million dollars.[1]

After a single one-hour visit, I walked out of her office free of pain and have not suffered a recurrence in the last 20 years.

The following day, enjoying my renewed sense of well-being, I went grocery shopping at my favorite health food store. The store was owned by Mr. Fritz, a gentleman in his 80s who was in glowing health. Since he had not seen me for quite a while, he inquired about my absence. I told him my story and explained that, as a result of my experience, I had been reading about the colon. This had led me to information about acidophilus and the importance of replacing this natural flora in my colon.

I told Mr. Fritz that, while I wanted to use acidophilus, I was uncertain as to which strain would be most effective. He told me that a human-strain acidophilus was essential for colon health, but that it would have no effect if taken orally. It needed to be implanted rectally, directly into the colon, for results. Since I seemed so interested, Mr. Fritz offered to give me a rare manuscript, suggesting it would answer my questions about acidophilus and reveal both the cause of my problem and the solution. Thus, I was introduced to the writings of James Empringham, Ph.D., Doctor of Science, which provided the inspiration and foundation for my future work and research.

Following Mr. Fritz's advice and the information in Dr. Empringham's book, I performed my first colon implant of acidophilus on myself. Immediately, I felt more overall energy and well-being.

Mr. Fritz attributed his years of excellent health to having a balanced colon flora. He recommended I write a book based on Dr. Empringham's work so this valuable information, which otherwise would be lost, could be made available to the public.

Feeling inspired, I set out to study the topic of colon health. Five years later, after researching all the citations found in medical library data banks, I realized that the knowledge imparted to me was not documented in the literature of the healing arts. Although evidence did point in this direction, it had never been compiled into one focused approach. For many years, I have felt a responsibility to my mentors to share this information with those suffering from chronic degenerative disease and with those studying the origin of such diseases.

It has been 20 years since I set foot on this unexpected avenue in my life. I followed Mr. Fritz's advice, and my booklet *Acidophilus & Colon Health* has been a steady seller since it was first published in 1980. The booklet has been updated several times as I have continued to gather a wealth of information. I applied this research in a practical manner and have gained six years of clinical experience.

Interest in my work and knowledge has grown. The climate and times are now ripe for this expanded, in-depth survey. There is a decline in health today due to environmental and dietary factors and overuse of antibiotics and other medications. This work provides the missing link to regaining the health of our immune system.

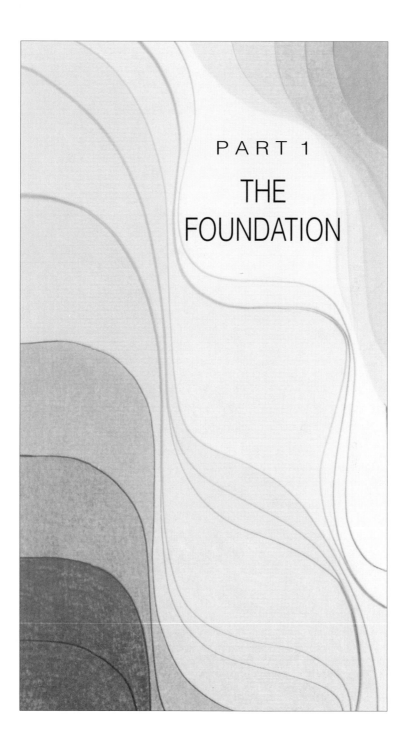

PART 1

THE
FOUNDATION

CHAPTER 1

In the Beginning

Time began. Atom, molecule, cell, and bacterium followed. Diversification progressed. Plants, fish, birds, reptiles, mammals, and human beings evolved.

From the darkness in the womb to the light of day, a baby is born and receives the first breath of life in the atmosphere. From our first taste of mother's milk to our last breath, the normal colon flora is absolutely essential for our survival throughout life.

Let us consider our beginning on earth. At birth, breast milk provides an infant the foundation necessary to form a strong immune system for life. In the first few days of life, breast milk is the link that extends mother's immunity to the infant. The antibodies in mother's milk offer the infant protection against the microorganisms capable of producing disease.

In addition to antibodies, all mammals receive an initial culture of beneficial bacteria from their mother's breast milk. Usually within the first few days of breastfeeding, the colon of a breastfed infant contains about 99% *Bifidobacterium bifidum*. Other bacteria, such as enterococci and coliform, constitute about 1% of the colon population.[1,2]

This absence of putrefactive bacteria is due to the slightly acid pH, which, in turn, is due to the predominance of *Bifidobacterium bifidum*. *B. bifidum* requires a slightly acidic medium for survival and also creates this slightly acidic pH as a result of its own metabolic activity of fermenting the milk sugar, lactose.[3] *B. bifidum* flourishes primarily on the high level of lactose and other nutrients contained in breast milk.[4]

Thus, the breastfed infant begins life with a good foundation of health and immunity built upon a beneficial colon flora implanted by the mother.

Lactobacteria Defined

The beneficial colon flora consists of several bacterial species. The most well-known, important species are *Lactobacillus acidophilus* and *Bifidobacterium bifidum*, though there are also other beneficial species. Since research indicates a healthy colon flora should contain a high percentage of *Lactobacillus acidophilus*, for the sake of simplicity, I am using the general term "lactobacteria" throughout this book to refer to the natural beneficial colon flora. Scientific names will be used when discussing a specific bacterium only.

The prefix "lacto-" is from the Latin word "lac," which means "milk." This refers to two significant features of lactobacteria. They convert carbohydrates to lactic acid in the colon through the process of fermentation. Second, the primary carbohydrate that lactobacteria ferment is lactose, or milk sugar.

Foundation of Health

A population of 99% *B. bifidum* in the breastfed infant is referred to as a "simplified flora," since one bacterium is so clearly the major constituent of the flora. As breastfed infants are weaned and introduced to a regular diet, their flora changes. Most notably, the *B. bifidum* content decreases in the colon. *Lactobacillus acidophilus* becomes prevalent, and other species take up residence as well. This condition is called a "mixed flora" and is considered normal as long as the beneficial lactobacteria make up about 80% of the colon population.

Similar to the flora of adults, the colon flora of bottle-fed infants is mixed and contains many unnecessary species of bacteria, fewer lactobacteria, and little, if any, *B. bifidum*.[5] Formula-fed infants are more susceptible to irritability, colic, and infection. This, in turn, leads to the inevitable use of antibiotics, resulting in a weakened immune system.[6]

When infants consume formulas made from cow's milk during

their first year of life, an allergic response can be triggered that will affect their gastrointestinal tract, lungs, blood, and skin. During breastfeeding, infants are less likely to experience allergies or asthma than bottle-fed babies.[7] In fact, 25% of infants who are allergic to cow's milk are also allergic to soy, which is the component commonly used in alternatives to cow's milk formulas. Since antigenically intact milk protein passes into breast milk, mothers who breastfeed their infants need to avoid excessive milk consumption.

When breastfeeding is not possible, some experts advise mothers to feed their infants hydrolyzed whey formula to avoid the allergic response to milk protein and soy.[8] Goat's milk is another alternative worth considering. Of course, a physician should always be consulted as to which formula is appropriate for an infant.

There are many excellent reasons for women to breastfeed their infants. Current research shows that a mother who nurses her baby for longer than four to six months is 49% less likely to develop breast cancer.[9] Breastfeeding fosters a nurturing bond between mother and infant. In addition, it provides the nutrient and bacterial foundation for a strong immune system. A recent study showed a correlation between breastfeeding and decreased incidence of otitis media (an ear infection). The risk of ear infection was significantly decreased in 289 children up to four months after breastfeeding was discontinued.[10]

When the protective flora is implanted in the infant's colon at birth and maintained throughout life, it contributes to sustained health.

Key to Health: The Colon

The colon is much more than an organ of elimination. It is a significant digestive organ. Important nutrients such as electrolytes and vitamins are absorbed into the body from the colon. Vitamin K and several B vitamins are manufactured by the lactobacteria that benefit us, the hosts.

The bacterial population of the colon determines the health of the colon, directly affecting other areas of the body. Substances in the

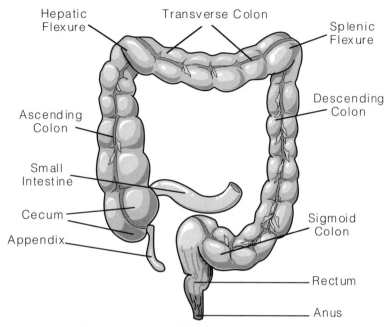

Figure 1. Colon Anatomy

colon are transported to the liver through the mesenteric and portal veins. From here, these substances can travel to the rest of the body via the bloodstream.

The colon flora plays a key role as part of the immune system in both infants and adults. The colon lactobacteria provide one of nature's first lines of defense in our bodies against invading microorganisms. When lactobacteria are established in the colon, disease-forming, opportunistic organisms are unable to take hold or survive. Lactobacteria literally provide a protective shield that constitutes a major aspect of our immune function.

The colon is the soil of the body. The natural lactobacteria colon flora represent the flowers growing in healthy soil. The pathogens (disease-producing microorganisms) represent the weeds that proliferate in unhealthy soil. Cultivating a healthy colon flora can be referred to as "intestinal gardening," a term first used by Dr. James Empringham. The analogy fits quite well.

Despite the scientific and technological advancements in medicine today, many Americans are not healthy. While modern medicine excels in emergency care, it lacks a holistic perspective and a truly preventive approach to illness. Fighting diseases and germs is not enough. We must return to the basic laws governing good health and, by applying these laws, learn how to optimize our well-being on all levels.

It is not enough to have anatomical knowledge of bodily functions. It is necessary to study and understand the interrelationship and interaction of all bodily systems and how these interactions influence our immunity and health.

The premise of my work is that the lactobacteria colon flora provide the foundation upon which life can thrive. With this foundation in place, good health and immunity can flourish, longevity can be realized. This is our birthright, a bacterial gift from nature. Before we can address the issue of disease, we must understand the importance of a balanced colon flora. This perspective brings fresh awareness.

When lactobacteria are predominant in the colon, maintaining the colon at a slightly acidic pH, we can achieve maximum health. This knowledge about the colon and its flora is the missing link in the practice of medicine and holistic health. By establishing and maintaining a slightly acidic colon environment in which harmful bacteria are unable to grow, much suffering and disease can be prevented.

Currently, there are many factors undermining this foundation. We will see how this gift, given to us by nature in the beginning, has been damaged and how we can restore this foundation of health. Once we understand the colon's role in health, immunity, and longevity, we can appreciate the profound potential of a scientifically based method for restoring the colon to its natural state.

There is a simple and direct path that leads to health. Reading this book can be the first step on such a journey. Times are changing, and time takes care of all things.

CHAPTER 2

The Protective Shield: Immunity and the Colon

When the first implant of beneficial bacteria is supplied by human breast milk at birth, growth factors and nutrients contained in mother's milk sustain its viability. After infancy, the implant can be maintained throughout life by correct diet, which includes consuming cultured-milk products containing lactose, the disaccharide sugar present in milk.

Each of us is inhabited by trillions upon trillions of microbes, both on our skin surface and within our bodies. At adulthood, the colon contains a vital life-support system of approximately 2.2 pounds of bacteria.[1] Some microorganisms produce harmful substances known as toxins. The capacity of a microorganism to produce toxins and the potency of the toxin are significant factors in the microbe's ability to cause disease.

Many people have pondered the fundamental question of why we, as a species, do not become extinct, since we are internally and externally bombarded by bacteria. One reason for our survival is that we have a mutually supportive relationship with some of these microbes. This is known as a "symbiotic" relationship. We provide them with a place of habitation and they, in turn, provide us with certain beneficial by-products.

This is clearly the case with the lactobacteria colon flora. The colon flora produce valuable nutrients that are assimilated into our body, and their slightly acidic secretions act as a barrier to prevent harmful microbes, parasites, or other pathogens from taking hold. This barrier is related to the important chemical variable known as pH.

Foundation of Life

When an architect designs a blueprint for a building, the plans must provide for a strong foundation. The foundation or substrate of all life on this planet is regulated by pH, which is the acid/alkaline balance.

A good gardener addresses the requirement for a strong foundation. Soil pH is the foundation that is essential for successful germination and healthy plant growth. A tree in unhealthy soil becomes an unhealthy tree, suffering disease and degeneration unless the soil is reestablished. In order to achieve lasting health, the tree cannot be symptomatically treated. It will only thrive when the soil is revitalized and conditions exist to support its growth.

The term "pH" is a chemical one, referring to the concentration of hydrogen ions in a solution. The higher the concentration of ions, the more active and "acidic" the solution. Solutions with a lower concentration of hydrogen ions are called "alkaline." This range of pH, from acid to alkaline, is measured from 0 to 14. A measurement of 7 indicates a neutral pH and is called a buffer, as it is neither acid nor alkaline. Each pH change of 1 on the scale reflects a tenfold increase. Thus, a substance with a pH of 1 is 10 times more acidic than a substance with a pH of 2.

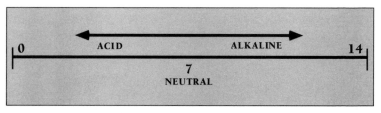

Figure 2. Basic pH Chart

At the cellular level, this activity of hydrogen ions in a solution (measured as pH) is the very basis of metabolic activity in our bodies. Every aspect of the body functions within a specific pH range. Outside of that range, disease, infection, malfunction, and even immediate death can result.

In health, the pH of the blood, extracellular fluid, and lower small

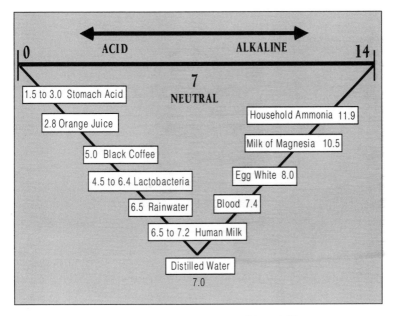

Figure 3. Substance pH Chart[3,4,5]

intestine should be alkaline. The pH of the saliva, stomach, urine, colon, and skin should be acidic.

Extracellular fluid bathes all the cells in our body. In health, this fluid is slightly alkaline, in the range of 7.35 to 7.45. Life can exist when the extracellular fluid is in the pH range of 6.8 to 7.8, but these are the outer limits.

Blood pH should be in the range of 7.35 to 7.45. If it becomes just a little too acidic, life-threatening conditions will follow. Blood that is too alkaline can also cause problems.

The stomach contains strong acids to prevent food from spoiling in the body, to kill harmful bacteria and other pathogens, and to digest components of our food. Stomach pH ranges from 1.5 (very acidic) to 3.0 (medium acidic), depending on the stomach's stage of digestion or rest.[2] When too little acid is produced in the stomach, digestion is hampered. When acid production is high, the lining of the stomach will be eaten away over time, resulting in ulcers.

These few examples illustrate the fine-tuning of our bodies' pH.

Homeostasis

"Homeostasis," the tendency toward equilibrium, is a survival mechanism of the body. No matter what our lifestyle or health habits, the body strives to maintain all functions necessary for life. Homeostasis is a compensatory function, which adjusts to inner and outer conditions as necessary. Thus, the body will function and maintain some outer semblance of health even under less-than-optimal conditions.

People with poor digestion or even those suffering from alcoholism often appear healthy for many years. The body will compensate up to a point, but it does operate within certain limits. The blood will not tolerate even minute changes in pH without dramatic effects. Other tissues or organs will tolerate greater deviations in pH for varying amounts of time. A change in the urine's pH can manifest quickly as a urinary tract infection, while a change in the stomach's pH takes much longer to show results. A person may have an insufficient concentration of hydrochloric acid in the stomach for years, but because this condition does not result in an immediate infection that demands attention, the person might suffer the results of improper digestion in the long run.

The colon has no sensory nerves, as have other areas of the body, to alert us of immediate problems. A colon condition will reach a severe state before becoming noticeable. The effect of an incorrect colon pH is a quiet but insidious contributor to disease. For maximum health, bodily functions must be optimized and the pH be addressed.

Digestion and pH

As we eat, we consume not only food but also multitudes of microbial species. The digestive system is divided into two major areas of function: the alimentary canal (the mouth, pharynx, esophagus, stomach, small intestine, and large intestine) and the accessory glands (salivary glands, liver, and pancreas).

The organs of the digestive system act on ingested food, enabling it to be utilized by the body as nutrients. In addition, our entire digestive tract, or alimentary canal, is equipped with features specifically designed to prevent harmful microbes, parasites, or other pathogens from establishing residence.

Digestion starts in the mouth, where pH level and bacterial content are just as important as elsewhere in the body. Bacteria or plaque growing on teeth can upset the microbial balance in the mouth, contributing to tooth decay and other oral ailments. As dentists know, microbes can gain entrance into the bloodstream quite easily through the mouth. Because harmful bacteria from the mouth can find their way to the heart and cause serious infection, people who have had rheumatic fever are required to take antibiotics prior to undergoing any dental procedures. If the mouth and saliva are healthy, many microbes will not be able to pass through our mouth, this outermost barrier.

After a short trip down the esophagus, the food and microbes encounter the stomach. Most microbial species are destroyed by the strong acid secretions of the stomach.[6] Putrefactive bacteria are inert in acid.

In 1865, Joseph Lister, the renowned British surgeon, found that diluted carbolic acid destroyed bacteria and prevented wounds and incisions from becoming infectious.[7] This is an example of how a strong acid solution will kill virulent bacteria.

Digestion and absorption of nutrients continues in the small intestine. From the ileum, the last section of the small intestine, digestive material enters the cecum, which is the beginning of the colon. In the colon, an acid pH prevents activation of harmful microorganisms, while an alkaline pH allows them to begin their work, breaking down dead, decaying organic matter and excreting toxic by-products.

Colon pH and Health

The single most important factor affecting colon pH is the type of bacteria that inhabits the colon. Research shows a direct correlation between lactobacteria flora in the colon and status of health. Those individuals who have a deficient flora tend to be less healthy. If the normal flora and slightly acid pH remained constant in the adult colon, would many degenerative conditions such as arthritis, neuritis, bursitis, colitis, and diverticulitis be prevented? This is, in fact, suggested by studies conducted over the last century.[8,9,10,11,12]

To prevent degenerative conditions in the human body, the correct acid pH (between 5.6 and 6.9) must be established in the colon and maintained for life. Then health must be sustained with nutrients and activity. Yet *Taber's Medical Dictionary* states that for the adult, the normal pH of the stool is neutral or slightly alkaline; for the infant, the normal pH is usually acid.[13]

Why does this contradiction in pH exist between infants and adults? Because average adults have lost most, if not all, of their initial lactobacteria implant received as infants. As we saw in the first chapter, the breastfed infant's colon contains about 99% *B. bifidum*. This bacterium specifically ferments carbohydrates and produces acids as by-products, which is why the healthy infant's colon and stool pH is slightly acidic. In good health, the pH of the adult colon and stool should also be slightly acidic.

An unfortunate fact of medical science is the way it determines what is a "normal" reading for lab results, such as blood or stool analysis. An average is calculated from all readings over a recent period and then defined as "normal." The figures used as guidelines reflect an average of the readings from unhealthy people! There are no figures reflecting what the reading should be for an optimally functioning, healthy person.

This situation needs to be remedied. Optimum health is our goal. Hence, while an alkaline stool pH might be common in adults today, it is not normal in a state of optimal health.

Although the category of lactobacteria is comprised of many species, most are similar in their ability to produce lactic acid.[14] This distinguishes them from the nonfermenting types of bacteria. We are concerned with the two species that are predominant in the healthy colon, *Lactobacillus acidophilus* and *Bifidobacterium bifidum*. Both are nonpathogenic, rod-shaped bacteria that produce mild acids from carbohydrates.[15,16] These lactobacteria ferment carbohydrates, espe-

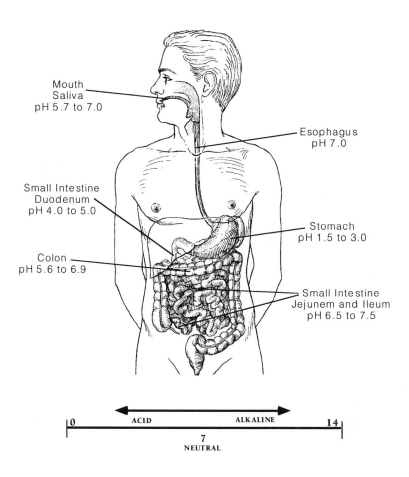

Mouth
Saliva
pH 5.7 to 7.0

Esophagus
pH 7.0

Small Intestine
Duodenum
pH 4.0 to 5.0

Stomach
pH 1.5 to 3.0

Colon
pH 5.6 to 6.9

Small Intestine
Jejunem and Ileum
pH 6.5 to 7.5

0   ACID   ALKALINE   14

7
NEUTRAL

Figure 4. pH of the Digestive Tract in Health

cially lactose (milk sugar), creating the metabolic by-product lactic acid along with small amounts of other acids, such as acetic acid.

This acid production is very significant. It is quite interesting that the lactobacteria produce the slightly acidic pH they require to thrive. They make the very environment they need.

Even the name of one of the main inhabitants of the healthy colon, *Lactobacillus acidophilus*, gives us pertinent information. "Acidophilus" means "acid loving." All lactobacteria are acid-producing and thrive only in slightly acidic environments. Would they be the main inhabitant of the colon if it were alkaline? Would the colon be alkaline in health with 80% colonization of lactobacteria? Certainly not.

The colon is the largest reservoir of microbes in the body, with 90% of the total fecal material in the colon containing bacteria.[17] When beneficial, acid-producing types of bacteria dominate the entire colon, including the interior wall of the colon, there is no room for foodborne pathogens to germinate and produce toxins.[18] Every container has a maximum capacity. In a garden with healthy soil, there is not enough room for weeds to grow.

Many scientists have noted that pathogenic bacteria and the majority of parasites can only live in an alkaline pH. They are unable to establish themselves and thrive in a slightly acidic pH. The layers of acid-producing lactobacteria that line the healthy colon form a protective shield of bacterial flora in the colon, making it impossible for pathogenic bacteria and parasites to take hold and penetrate the colon lining.

The colon must be restored to its natural state. It is meant to be a fermentation chamber, colonized by at least 80% lactobacteria that are all happily producing the very slightly acidic secretions needed to support their life and proliferation. A slightly acidic colon pH is the essential foundation for maximum health. This fact will help set the record straight to clear and resolve the confusion that prevails today.

CHAPTER 3

A Crisis in Health Care: The Neglected Colon

Over the last 100 years, with the growth of industrialization, many factors have contributed to the breakdown of our natural colon flora defense system, allowing the invasion of harmful microorganisms and parasites. Not long ago, country doctors assisted women with home births. Grandmothers taught breastfeeding, gave enemas when needed, and offered fresh lemon juice and freshly-picked herbal remedies for the common cold. Why have we abandoned this simple, healthy way of life?

In the 1890s, new technology led to the discovery of chemical isolates, enabling synthetic drugs to be produced. The age of modern medications began.

One specific group of drugs has well-known adverse effects on the lactobacteria colon flora. In the 1940s, antibiotics, the new "magic bullets," became the focus of modern medicine. While health professionals as far back as 1950 recognized that antibiotics destroy the lactobacteria flora in the colon, no effective steps were taken to replenish this natural flora after a course of antibiotics was completed. New health problems have become widespread in great part because a method to replace the damaged colon flora has not been incorporated into the health care process.

Used correctly, antibiotics save lives. However, a post-antibiotic therapy must be administered in order to recolonize the beneficial bacteria that provide the foundation for good health in our body.

Modern medicine has missed the essential step of restoring balance following a course of antibiotics. Even today, few understand that replacing the natural lactobacteria flora cannot be accomplished by oral consumption of any lactobacteria product.

Deterioration of Our Protective Shield

Antibiotics kill bacteria without differentiating between harmful and beneficial types. After a course of antibiotics, the colon flora is severely damaged. Since the lactobacteria flora is no longer predominant, the colon pH is no longer slightly acidic. When alkaline, the colon is perfect terrain for growth of pathogenic microorganisms. These life forms can take hold and become a source of many toxic metabolic by-products that directly or indirectly harm the human immune system.

Misuse of antibiotics is analogous to tending a garden by using a shovel to turn the soil to get rid of the weeds but forgetting to fertilize the soil and to plant seeds. In this scenario, planting ground cover, flowers, or crops is neglected and weeds proliferate even more vigorously than before. Nothing has been established in the garden that will grow and inhibit the weeds.

No one would keep repeating this inefficient procedure, yet that is exactly what is happening in the human colon today. The gardeners are not educated as to the proper care of their own soil.

Medicine has been battling these microorganisms for many years. Direct attack with antibiotics and other frontline medicines was effective for nearly 40 years, from the 1940s into the 1980s. Currently, we are losing the battle. A fresh approach — indeed, a whole new view is necessary.

The early 1900s brought dramatic changes in the food-processing industry. Liquid and hydrogenated vegetable oils were manufactured by a process requiring the use of harsh chemicals and high temperatures. Modern research shows the dangers of these hydrogenated and processed oils that have been consumed in large quantities only in this century.[1] Convenience foods, devitalized from processing methods and long shelf lives, have become a way of life in the 20th century. As an outgrowth of the coal tar and nerve gas industries, pesticides were manufactured and entered the food chain. Last, but not least, alcohol and tobacco have been commonly used and abused in this century. The adverse effects of these and other drugs on health is well documented.

These dietary changes, initiated during the early 1900s, combined with environmental and medical factors, have damaged our natural lactobacteria colon flora. How can we be assured that our lack of beneficial flora will be corrected? This question will be answered by linking experience with many avenues of historical and recent research that regard the colon and its flora as part of a whole system. Although the significance of this valuable flora is generally overlooked, it is a critical part of our immune system and has a tremendous impact on our health and longevity.

The holistic perspective includes knowledge of colon function and ecology, the relationship of the colon to other organs, and the role of the colon in human health. It is my hope that further research will be initiated in this vital area.

Before we examine how to reestablish the colon as a key to our health, we will explore some of the causes and effects of the damaged colon lactobacteria.

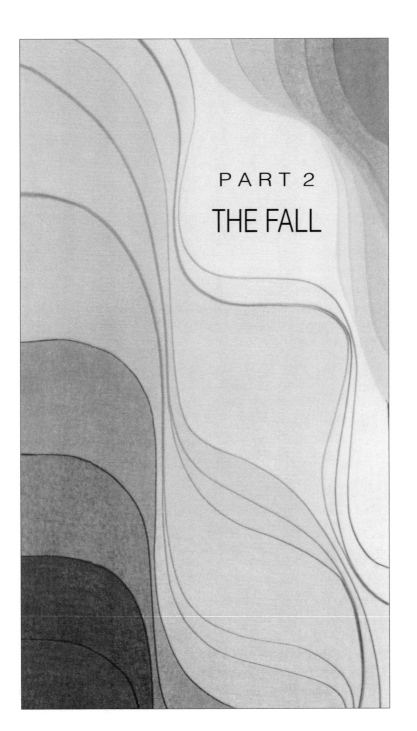

PART 2

THE FALL

CHAPTER 4

The War: The Visible Army Versus the Invisible Army

Two armies are at war, one visible and the other invisible. The visible army is one part of nature, representing the total human population of the world, either 5 billion strong or 5 billion weak, depending on your view. The invisible army, another part of nature, represents the overwhelming numbers of organisms that have established their stronghold long before the visible army arrived. As mere sojourners in space passing through a fleeting existence, we, the visible army, should show respect for all life.

In 1940, Phase I began. The visible army started a war, an attempt to fight infections caused by the invisible army of microorganisms. The visible army's weapon was penicillin, which destroyed some pathogenic troops when it entered the scene.

The unseen war progressed, and troop movement was observed only by scientists looking through microscopes. During these initial years, GREEN lights were on, and more antibiotics were being readied as a back-up arsenal.

In the 1970s, Phase II began, and the ORANGE light switched on: PROCEED WITH CAUTION. The invisible army was not resting and had not rested since the natural balance was upset in 1940. The microcosm continued to adjust by preparing for an all-out war and was largely undisturbed by the initially lost battle.

One night, an unknown microorganism that had never been previously detected was isolated in the laboratory. Word went out to all concerned scientists on the front lines that a multidrug-resistant organism was no longer sensitive to penicillin!

Much to the surprise of the visible army, the tables have turned, and the microcosm is beginning to win the war. Microorganisms are becoming increasingly resistant to the antibiotic arsenal.

Is there a way to enact a truce before these minute microorganisms annihilate the human population? Today, the most agile minds on this planet have started to switch on the RED lights: DANGER!

We, the visible army, are completely unaware that the invisible microcosm is a vital, integral part of ourselves. The microcosm is necessary for the biological functioning of all mammals from birth until death. For the most part, we have destroyed our major line of protection, the colon lactobacteria, with the very artillery of antibiotics that was intended to save us. Our protection is being lost to an invisible enemy who has advanced beyond our borders and has started to degrade our immune system from within! Now, the way is made much easier for outside invaders to enter and gain their foothold in the human system.

The Invaders

Force 1. Bacteria

From the discovery of penicillin came the weapon of antibiotics, targeted against pathogens. The purpose of the weapon was to destroy the pathogen's ground troops as quickly as possible. Pathogens use their volatile, poisonous metabolic by-products as ammunition and flourish in the endless food supplied by putrefaction in the abnormal human colon. The ammunition acts through slow absorption into the human system and weakens the host's immunity, setting the stage for invasion by harmful microorganisms.

Force 2. Yeast/Fungi

These opportunists rank close behind the pathogens. They are the undercover reinforcements for the pathogens, waiting in the trenches for the lactobacteria forces in the colon to be destroyed. As the opportunists continue to rise, the yeast and fungi begin to hit harder and faster and gain a further stronghold in the colon.

For ammunition, the opportunists use gas attacks, a result of their production of acetaldehyde and other metabolic by-products, further degrading human health. Their primary food supply includes sugar, vinegar, wine, and yeast. In today's chemical warfare, when pushed back and suppressed, yeast and fungi have a remarkable capacity to change, and are extremely difficult to eradicate. Once established, they are well prepared for a long battle, to the detriment of the immune system.

Force 3. Parasites

After the lactobacteria are wiped out and the colon is secured by Forces 1 and 2, the parasites can now conquer. Parasites are ubiquitous and have fought wars since the beginning of time. Their medium is primarily the abnormal, putrefactive, alkaline pH condition that is present in the average human colon today. The stage is set, the ground troops are in place, and the situation can escalate even further. The host begins to succumb to the toxic combinations seeping into the interior of his or her body.

Some types of parasites have an airborne division capable of entering the human body through the lungs. Other types gain entry into the human body by riding on food as a means of transportation. Parasites strive to remain undetected in their host's gastrointestinal tract. They are masters of deception, mimic many diseases, use camouflage, and can often evade the most sophisticated equipment. They are almost impossible to destroy completely because they produce thousands of invisible reproductive eggs.

The human opposition forces that seek to destroy them use very strong antiparasitic drugs. Some of these drugs constitute a cure that may be harder on the host than on the parasite they are intended to destroy.

Force 4. Viruses

Last to enter the battleground are viruses, the real destroyers of life. These organisms are the elite, small, hardy, and difficult to control, let alone destroy.

These are the dangerous armies of the microcosm. Once bacteria, yeast/fungi, and parasites have taken over the human body, decomposition begins while the host still breathes. At some point, autoimmune disease overwhelms the host and homeostasis ends. The war is over for that individual, who has been destroyed from within.

However, there are also many beneficial microorganisms. The question is one of proper balance. This interplay is perhaps most evident in the human colon, where the relationship between the microcosm of beneficial bacteria and human physiology is essential to our health. As long as beneficial microorganisms are in the majority, comprising at least 80% of the population in the colon, harmony reigns. It is only when harmful microorganisms gain the upper hand that chaos and devastation of health ensue.

Fighting these invaders directly has only made them stronger. Through their capacity for rapid mutation, bacteria, viruses, and even parasites are now resistant to modern drugs. Our current arsenal of antibiotics is no longer effective.[1,2,3,4,5]

In order to survive, the human race must coexist with the microcosm. If we annihilate bacteria, yeast, fungi, parasites, and viruses, the human race will cease to exist. Since the beginning of time, this has been the law.

We must pool all available resources to find effective solutions without creating more imbalance. It is time to end the war and explore new avenues for answers.

The alternative approach, which must now be taken, is to increase host resistance to these invaders. When the body no longer provides fertile soil for harmful microorganisms, and the immune system is strong, balance can be restored.

CHAPTER 5

Antibiotics: Defense Betrayed

Nature intended microorganisms and humans to evolve in unison. Life and death are dependent on bacterial support. Although we live harmoniously with many microorganisms, others are lethal and threaten our very existence.

Our thrust to combat the force of aggressive microbes began in the 1890s, when new information was discovered in the field of microbiology. In 1889, Vuillemin described "antibiosis," the process whereby one microorganism destroys the life of another in order to sustain its own life.[1]

In 1924, Gratia and Dath discovered the antibiotic actinomycetin, produced from strains of actinomycetes soil organisms.[2] Sir Alexander Fleming, a Scottish bacteriologist and physician, observed in 1929 that an agar plate inoculated with *Staphylococcus aureus* had become contaminated with a mold colony. A clear zone surrounded the mold colony, indicating inhibition of bacterial growth. He then identified the mold and studied its antibacterial activities.[3] Since 1940, a number of antibiotics have been created from the microorganisms discovered by these men.

During World War II, penicillin became the magic bullet and thousands of lives were saved from the scourge of bacteria-related infections. Between 1940 and 1970, an increasing number of new antibiotics were introduced, giving the public a sense of safety and security.

From this newfound infatuation with antibiotics, the industry grew to its current proportion, with annual production in the United States currently equal to 40 million pounds.[4]

The Research Train: Faster Than a Speeding Bullet

In evolutionary terms, microorganisms predate life as we know it. Microorganisms adjusted and evolved along with the evolving earth and plant and animal kingdoms. Now, they are adjusting to every imaginable chemical produced by man. Researchers are currently under pressure to win the war by producing new drugs in a race to keep up with the incredibly fast mutation rate of microbes. Although guided by the results seen in the microscope and the test tube, scientists in the laboratory cannot always predict what will happen in a living system.

The research train is speeding in order to develop more effective antibiotics. However, even when new antibiotics are developed, they will not emerge from the Food and Drug Administration's (FDA) review process for at least 10 years. In that period, the new antibiotic risks obsolescence before it can be used. Stop a moment to consider the long-range effects of this fact on the world population.

In a mere 30-year period, bacteria have become increasingly resistant to our antibiotic arsenal. In his book, *The Antibiotic Paradox,* Stuart Levy, M.D., eloquently describes the results of our naive overuse of antibiotics. Dr. Levy, professor of medicine, molecular biology, and microbiology at Tufts University School of Medicine, is recognized as the leading international expert on antibiotic use and resistance. He discovered the mechanism for tetracycline resistance and was first to document the transfer of multidrug resistance between animals and humans.

Dr. Levy describes the ability of bacteria to convey drug resistance information among each other and even to dissimilar species. This is now occurring at an increasing rate. Resistance genes that were first identified in Gram-positive bacteria have been located in Gram-negative bacteria. Aerobic and anaerobic types of microorganisms are now exchanging genetic material.

This free exchange of antibiotic-resistance genes between bacterial species is beginning to have a devastating impact on our health. Penicillin is currently ineffective against many strains of gonorrhea found worldwide. In Africa, 50% of the causative bacteria for cholera are resistant to tetracycline.[5] Tuberculosis is back with a vengeance, with new strains completely resistant to most available antibiotics. Difficult-to-treat or lingering ear infections in children are becoming more common. Antibiotics are not as successful in treating these ear infections as they previously were, and children are sometimes kept on antibiotics for years because no lasting results are achieved.

In 1994, we were stunned by Dr. Levy's report that antibiotics were no longer the magic bullet. Dr. Levy's urgent message to the world cannot be ignored. The rate of adaptation by bacteria far exceeds both the rate of human adaptation and the rate of human technological advances. In his book, Dr. Levy cites many examples of multidrug resistance and their mechanisms.

Antibiotic resistance can be triggered several ways. In the early 1800s, mercury was first used for amalgam dental fillings because medical authorities believed that mercury would not be released into the body. However, in the 1980s, a research team observed that mercury caused bacteria to become antibiotic resistant. In 1993, a study of 640 individuals at the University of Georgia, Athens indicated that amalgam tooth fillings were a contributing factor to antibiotic resistance. The fillings were releasing mercury; contact with mercury causes genetic changes in human oral and intestinal bacteria. Those bacteria that are not destroyed by mercury acquire genetic resistance to the toxicity of mercury.[6]

We can no longer think in terms of combating individual microorganisms. As a result of their rapid information exchange, microorganisms now exist as a totality of diverse types.[7]

An experiment was performed in an agricultural setting that illustrates just how rapidly microorganisms exchange information. Baby chicks were hatched and then given feed laced with oxytetracycline. The *Escherichia coli* bacteria in the feces of the chicks were monitored. Within a mere 24 to 36 hours, strains of *E. coli*, resistant to oxytetracycline, were isolated from the chicks. These strains had also developed resistance to antibiotics not even used on the farm.

The stools of the farmers themselves were examined over a period of five to six months. The surprise was that farm workers and their families, living 200 feet away from these oxytetracycline-fed chicks, showed the same change in their *E. coli*. Although the farmers and their families were neither taking antibiotics nor eating the chickens, their *E. coli* also developed resistance to oxytetracycline.[8]

This study is just one illustration of how overusing an antibiotic leads to resistance to many antibiotics. The remarkable fact is that this resistance is transmitted between bacteria and across species. Even people who have not taken antibiotics are affected by antibiotic overuse in treating animals and humans. Such research has profound implications, especially when we consider this has all transpired just in the past 50 years.

The use of antibiotics in treating illness is a shotgun approach that destroys the beneficial flora along with the disease-forming bacteria. Our immune system has suffered as a result of that shotgun blast. Because microorganisms constantly readjust to their environment and become progressively multiresistant, physicians have prescribed increasingly stronger doses of antibiotics over time. This increase has annihilated our protective shield, the beneficial colon flora, provided by nature to humans at birth. Our entire immune system suffers defeat as we become deficient in our normal levels of beneficial flora.

Nature intended the friendly lactobacteria in the colon to be our frontline defense, an army of immune system protectors. Without this protection, we suffer. For every force, there is a counter-force. It seems that the microcosm of invisible microorganisms is the real master of planet earth. We have won the battle and are rapidly losing the war!

As a health researcher and professional colon hygienist, I have listened to numerous stories from men and women about their downward spiral of failing health. Overuse or misuse of antibiotics at some point in their lives is the common theme in these stories.

Before taking any medication, we must ask questions. Many people are treated with antibiotics even when the causative organism has not been identified. For example, the possibility of yeast infections in ears should be considered when antibiotics are not getting results.[9] Another example is congestion in the sinus cavity, which is commonly treated by antibiotic therapy. If the congestion is caused by anything other than a susceptible bacterial strain, the only thing accomplished by antibiotic therapy is creating a weakened immune system that will be more vulnerable to attack by multiresistant organisms in the near future. One result of a deteriorating immune system is the attack of white blood cells (lymphocytes) on one's own tissues, an autoimmune disease.

Stop the Train!

The research train started on the track 100 years ago. For every year it has been running, it has increased its speed one mile per hour. We are going so fast now that we can't see the forest for the trees! Before we create more problems for ourselves, let's take a short rest, gather our senses, and assess what is valid in the healing arts at present.

Is there enough time to return our immune system to where it was prior to the 1940s?

In 1970, at the University of Florida, Shands Teaching Hospital, 96% of the *Staphylococcus* strains analyzed proved to be sensitive to erythromycin. This sensitivity resulted from restricted use of erythromycin for three years. In parts of the nation where use of the drug had not been restricted, sensitivity to erythromycin was minimal. Simply restricting the use of the antibiotic for three years allowed it to again be useful against *Staphylococcus*.[10]

If this result is seen with one antibiotic, perhaps it would also be seen with other antibiotics that are no longer effective due to over-use. It certainly is worth a try in order to prevent the creation of multidrug-resistant strains in the future.

OK, start the train, but proceed with caution.

Following the judicious use of antibiotics, a post-antibiotic therapy is needed. Such treatment is necessary to replenish the normal colon flora, which will enable it to combat most foreign microorganisms. Post-antibiotic therapy restores a major part of the immune system to proper functional balance.

An effective method of post-antibiotic therapy is discussed in Part 4. Historically, no such post-antibiotic therapy has been applied. When antibiotic therapy destroys the resident lactobacteria of the colon, which are not replaced, the colon is then susceptible to the next line of aggressors: the pathogens, yeasts, parasites, and viruses.

CHAPTER 6

Candida

In the normal, healthy colon, yeasts are typically present at a ratio of one yeast per 1,000 lactobacteria. Present in this ratio, yeasts do no harm. However, when the colon flora becomes abnormal, this ratio reverses to become one lactobacterium per 1,000 yeast.[1] In losing the normal protective flora in our colon, we have become open territory for yeasts.[2] Yeasts are recognized to be man's most common pathogen, with 150 species isolated in different infections.[3]

The most common yeast culprit, responsible for many clinical syndromes, is *Candida albicans*. Although *Candida* usually does not enter the bloodstream, it secretes soluble metabolites that are absorbed through mucosal surfaces. When the normal flora is destroyed by antibiotics, birth control pills, or medications such as steroids, this opportunistic organism can overgrow the mucosal surfaces of the mouth, colon, and vagina. When it does enter the bloodstream, the resulting symptoms are collectively referred to as "polysystemic chronic candidiasis." [4]

Candida is known to cause thrush (*Candida* in the mouth), vulvovaginitis (associated with women's use of antibiotic therapy), balanitis (*Candida* infecting glands of the penis, transmitted during intercourse), and cystitis (inflammation of the bladder). Deep-organ candidiasis is a serious systemic multi-organ infection. It is prevalent in AIDS patients, cancer patients, and burn victims.

The Centers for Disease Control (CDC) do not record data on *C. albicans*, "...as it is not a communicable disease." This contradicts statements from other authorities, who describe *Candida albicans* as being transmitted by sexual contact, by hands of medical attendants, and from the colonized birth canal to the neonatal oropharynx.[5] *Can-*

dida albicans is one of the three most common organisms to be isolated from blood cultures in hospitals.[6]

A 1990 study of women with candidiasis hypersensitivity syndrome appeared in *The New England Journal of Medicine*. This article reported that nystatin did not reduce the psychological or systemic symptoms associated with the syndrome significantly more than the placebo.[7]

Lactobacillus acidophilus, part of the normal protective flora found in the vagina, is susceptible to the effects of antibiotic overuse. Women often develop vaginal *Candida* after antibiotic use. When vulvovaginitis caused by *Candida* is treated by a five- to seven-day course of nystatin, clotrimazole, miconazole, or butoconazole, relapse is common.[8] Both pharmaceutical and natural treatment modalities have the capacity for relapse if any yeast cells remain in the colon or vagina and the proper flora has not been established following treatment.

Correcting the colon flora alone may not eliminate *Candida* that has spread to other areas of the body. It is essential first to eliminate almost all the *Candida* from the system. Then the cause of *Candida* overgrowth must be corrected at the source, the colon. This prevents relapse through strengthening the whole system at the foundation. This is an important point.

In the health-conscious segment of society, many people know about yeast infections. However, people are sometimes diagnosed as having yeast infections without laboratory confirmation. While missing this critical confirmation of yeast overgrowth, these individuals are put on extreme diets to rid their system of yeast. Currently, there is an effective laboratory analysis that can determine if yeasts are present at pathogenic levels. Such an analysis is necessary to determine if *Candida* is actually the culprit.

By observing the growth requirements for culturing *C. albicans* in the laboratory, we see relationships emerge between *Candida* growth, lactobacteria growth, and the colon environment. When laboratory culture media is vitamin-deficient, *Candida* thrives. Lactobacteria, on the other hand, require specific nutrients, including riboflavin, niacin, pantothenate, pyridoxine, and others.[9] Thus, in the human body, a nutritious diet will support an existing healthy flora, and will be unfavorable for *Candida*.

In addition, the normal, slightly acidic colon flora produces vitamins such as niacin, thiamine, riboflavin, pyridoxine, folic acid, pantothenic acid, biotin, vitamin B_{12}, and vitamin K, which are utilized by the human host.[10] This further enhances the nutritional status, health, and immunity of the person.

In laboratory conditions, the population of yeasts is reduced when the pH is slightly acid, between 5.3 and 5.8. In the human body, the pH of the colon is maintained at an acidic level as a result of lactic acid and other acid secretions by the naturally occurring lactobacteria. Thus, when lactobacteria populate the colon, the pH is adverse for *C. albicans* reproduction.[11]

There can only be disease where there is a medium!

CHAPTER 7

Parasites:
Opportunistic Organisms

As we saw in the previous chapter, when the natural colon flora is disturbed, opportunistic organisms such as yeasts can establish themselves. Parasites are another class of opportunistic organisms. When an individual's immune system, saliva, stomach, and small intestine are healthy, and the colon flora supports the correct, slightly acidic pH, it is unlikely that parasites can become established.

By definition, parasites require the support of a host to sustain their existence. Generally, they cannot assimilate food directly and depend on predigested food from their host. The parasitic relationship is usually deleterious to the host without causing death to the host. In order for the parasite to flourish, the host must remain alive!

Parasitic disease can be chronic and cause many symptoms, few symptoms, or no symptoms at all. A carrier can be infectious without having an obvious infection. In these cases, a balance of sorts exists between the host and the parasite. Parasites can survive in low numbers and multiply rapidly when the host's resistance drops due to high stress, nutrient deficiency, trauma, and sudden or chronic illness. Some parasites once considered harmless are now a major cause of severe illness and even death in those who are chronically ill or who have autoimmune diseases.

Gender and age are not predisposing factors when it comes to parasitic infection. Initially, the patient may complain of constipation, diarrhea, irritable bowel syndrome, fatigue, edema, low back pain, sciatica, frequent nasal draining, and flatulence. Flatulence and bloating can be constant, increasing after meals. Other signs can include craving for food even after eating a meal, weight loss or gain, and iron-deficiency anemia.

Patients who suffer from these chronic conditions frequently seek help from a variety of therapeutic modalities and only experience temporary relief. In many cases, when treatments should have reached their peak effectiveness, relapse occurs and treatment is discontinued.

One possible indication of parasitic disease is frequency of elimination. For those individuals whose colon is eliminating more than two times a day, I recommend a stool analysis. Since parasites are translucent, they cannot be seen using x-ray technology. Fiber optics do not identify parasites, and incomplete fecal testing is worthless.

Modes of Infection

Parasites reach susceptible hosts from their primary sources through various methods. Some parasites require only direct contact. Others with more complicated life cycles pass through developmental stages, either as free-living forms or as intermediate hosts, before becoming infective. Transmission can take place directly from polluted water, food, soil, and from contact with infected animals or insects. Most developed nations have adequately addressed the primary source of transmission by providing good hygiene and sanitation.

Humans infected by parasites may either be (1) the only host, (2) the principal host with other humans also infected, or (3) the "incidental" host, where the parasite becomes established in a host it does not generally prefer.

Parasites have a worldwide distribution. Although tropical temperatures and humidity favor parasites, they also commonly occur in North America, Canada, Alaska, and Russia. Low temperatures usually prevent eggs and larvae from developing. Since moisture and warmth are essential for parasites, they are activated in the warm body of a host.

In the last few years, parasites have been causing much more trouble than ever before. Even as parasitic infections are on the rise, many people and health practitioners still consider parasites to be exclusively a Third World problem. This is not the case. As world population and air travel have increased, the distribution of parasites has become widespread. After traveling to places such as India, Bali, or South America, people return home to the United States feeling fine, only to become quite ill within a four-week period. This is the incubation time necessary for parasitic eggs to hatch!

Since parasites can be found on the best of high-quality produce in any household or restaurant, exercise caution when visiting open salad bars and restaurants offering fresh-squeezed vegetable juices. Because we cannot see contaminants on our food without the benefit of a microscope, we should always wash, scrape, and peel raw foods before eating them.

This sounds like common sense, but it is amazing how many people still eat food directly from the produce section of the supermarket or health food store without first washing it well. The label "organically grown" is meaningful to the consumer, but meaningless to the parasite. Parasites do not distinguish between organic and chemically treated foods.

Most parasites are destroyed at the temperatures achieved in ordinary cooking. Eating raw fish is gambling with your health. A fisherman opening a freshly caught fish and finding a belly full of worms is a sight you will never forget.

Worm larvae may exist even in the best quality of fish, but there is no way to confirm their presence without a microscope. Why take chances? Cook most of your foods, especially your fish!

If a patient's parasitic infection has been detected by laboratory analysis, pharmaceutical or natural remedies can be prescribed. However, treatment for such infections does not constitute a quick fix. The infected individual must comply with the course of treatment and follow fastidious hygiene practices. The house, toilets, bedding, and yard should be kept as clean as possible. Hands must be clean for food preparation and eating, and children should be instructed to wash their hands after going to the bathroom, petting animals, or participating in playground activities.

When I began to research the topic of parasites, I found the available reference material to be limited. I asked the reference librarian at a medical library why there were so few technical books on parasites. She replied, "Who wants to study parasites?"

Many people today may be indifferent or squeamish about the topic of parasites. However, the importance of the topic cannot be denied. I am presenting the following information so that we can all appreciate the far-reaching implications of the prevalence of parasitic infections.

Nematodes

The roundworm, or *Ascaris lumbricoides,* is similar to an earthworm in appearance and infects more people in the world than any other parasite. Twenty-two percent of the world population is estimated to be infected with this organism, with 1,550 annual deaths occurring from intestinal obstruction.[1] There are 500,000 species of this parasite. Approximately 18,000 tons of eggs are produced every year in China alone. These worms stretched head-to-tail would circle the world 50 times![2]

One female roundworm can produce 200,000 eggs per day. The adult worm lives in the upper small intestine where it consumes predigested food from its host.[3] Larvae hatch in the duodenum, penetrate the mucosal lining, and migrate to the lungs through the blood or lymph.[4] The first symptoms of infection mimic those of pneumonia: coughing, wheezing, and fever. When adult forms are coughed from the lungs to the mouth and swallowed, they are again introduced into the intestinal tract. Adult worms mature in the ileum within about nine weeks.[5]

The symptoms of this infection can range from weight loss to weight gain, unsatisfied hunger, water retention, odorous gas, bloating, bad breath, belching, environmental and/or food allergies, asthma, fatigue, insomnia, disorientation, and inability to digest gluten, the protein in wheat. Diarrhea, cramps, and intestinal obstruction occur in some people.[6] Mental and emotional symptoms may also be caused by these parasites. In preschool children, infection by nematodes can cause lactose intolerance, with a serious infection causing intestinal obstruction, vomiting, and abdominal tenderness.[7]

Trichuriasis trichiura, or whipworm, is another nematode. This parasite has a worldwide distribution, lives in the colon, and has been frequently reported as a cause of appendicitis.[8]

Perhaps the most well-known parasite in the United States is the pinworm. These are small, thread-like worms that cause rectal itching. Eggs can lodge under the fingernails and be transmitted through food handling, animals, and dirt.

Cestodes

When the beef tapeworm, or *Taenia saginata*, is established in an individual, it inhabits the small intestine. Instead of digesting food, the tapeworm absorbs food from the intestine of its host. It is transmitted by uncooked beef and pork.

The fish tapeworm, or *Diphyllobothrium latum,* is found in raw or undercooked fish and has a worldwide distribution. The presence of the adult worm in the human intestinal tract causes very few symptoms. The bodies of fish tapeworms are segmented and attach to the intestinal surface.[9] They may cause abdominal discomfort, a vitamin B_{12} deficiency, and anemia. Since these infections are not easy to treat, a physician who specializes in infectious diseases should be consulted. The head of the worm must be removed from the intestinal surface or it can establish itself again.

Tapeworm infections are found in Mexico, South America, Africa, Pakistan, Southeast Asia, China, and India. They were recently introduced to Irian Jaya via infected pigs from Bali. These populations now experience widespread infections.

Trematodes

These are commonly known as flukes. They are vertebrate parasites that are transmitted to humans through eating crabs, snails, or even prawns. There are also lung flukes and liver flukes.

The intestinal fluke *Fasciolopsis buski* is a giant trematode found in Taiwan, China, Vietnam, Thailand, Indonesia, Malaysia, and the Indian subcontinent. These flukes attach themselves to the duodenum and jejunum of the host and cause indigestion, diarrhea, abdominal pain, edema, and malabsorption. Raw or undercooked bamboo shoots and water chestnuts may be sources of infection.

Flagellates

Flagellates belong to the protozoan kingdom. One of the most widespread protozoans is *Giardia lamblia*. An estimated 200 million people are infected by *Giardia lamblia* worldwide, and the incidence of this infection is increasing.[10] This organism infests impure water and has been located in urban tap water, well water, and even pristine streams of the Rocky Mountains. During its life cycle, the organism forms cysts that are resistant to chlorine and spread by person-to-person transmission.[11] There have been outbreaks even in cities with chlorinated water. Water filters with a pore size of 0.5 microns exclude *Giardia*.

This flagellate invades the gallbladder, duodenum, and upper intestine, where it can reduce immunoglobulin A, our source of secretory antibodies. When symptomatic, it results in diarrhea, malabsorption, bloating, and weight loss. It usually takes several weeks to cause infection.[12]

Parasitic Infection Statistics

The following data is derived from a report by the World Health Organization (WHO). The report estimates annual rates of infection and death due to parasites from 1975 to 1989.[13] It is important to note that many areas of the world do not record this data; therefore, the actual numbers may be higher. All figures are for worldwide incidence.

Consequences of Parasitic Infections

Often, toxic drugs are the only treatment that will effectively kill parasites. Benefits versus risks must always be considered. Many rem-

Nematodes

Infestation	# Infected Per Year	# of Deaths Per Year
Lymphatic filariasis	85-100 million	none reported
Hookworm	900 million	none reported
Onchocerciasis	30 million	none reported
Strongyloidiasis	35 million	none reported
Dracunculiasis	10 million	none reported
Ascariasis (Roundworm)	1 billion	1,550
Trichostrongylosis	5.5 million	none reported
Trichuriasis (Whipworm)	500-800 million	none reported

Trematodes

Infestation	# Infected Per Year	# Of Deaths Per Year
Schistosomiasis	200 million	500,000 to 1 million
Paragonimiasis	3.2 million	none reported
Fasciolopsiasis	10 million	none reported
Clonorchiasis and Opisthorchiasis	19 million	none reported
Fasciolopsis buski	10 million	none reported

Cestode

Infestation	# Infected Per Year	# Of Deaths Per Year
Cestodiases (Tapeworm)	65 million	none reported

Protozoa

Infestation	# Infected Per Year	# Of Deaths Per Year
Amebiasis	50 million	40,000-110,000
American trypanosomiasis	24 million	60,000
African trypanosomiasis	100,000 million	5,000
Leishmaniasis	1.2 million	none reported
Malaria	400-490 million	2.2-2.5 million
Giardiasis	200 million	none reported

Table 1. Worldwide Parasitic Infection[14]

edies do not work because the parasites are either unidentified or identified incorrectly.

When parasites are correctly identified and destroyed, debris from the breakdown of the dead parasites will reach the colon. This debris must be removed from the colon in order to prevent relapse and further contamination of the system. This can be compared to weeding a garden. When a gardener destroys the weeds, he has to carry them away from the garden both to clear the garden of debris and to prevent the weeds from reestablishing themselves.

Even when the main site of infection by parasites is the small intestine, toxic metabolic end products eventually reach the colon. If the colon is already in an unhealthy state, these end products and decay will cause further problems. If the infection is massive, even the normal colon flora can be overwhelmed.

After the infection has been correctly diagnosed and the parasites have been destroyed, the colon should be cleansed promptly to remove any dead parasites and putrefaction. Then the natural flora must be immediately restored so the colon can regain its natural slightly acidic state and resume its normal function to protect against further infestation. In most cases, this will prevent relapse. In all cases, the cyclic nature of parasitic infestations should be considered in any treatment plan.

For more than 600 million years, parasites have been evolving with their host systems, and the survivors of these genetic changes remain with us today. By accepting the presence of parasites we can take scientific, practical steps to control them. In order to prevent parasitic infection, the host's resistance can be maintained and good hygiene practices should be followed. Prevention precedes cure!

CHAPTER 8

Bacterial Polluters

In August 1992, two farm workers died from exposure to hydrogen sulfide gas, asphyxiated when they entered manure waste pits. Anaerobic bacteria decompose manure, generating methane, hydrogen sulfide, carbon dioxide, and ammonia. These gases can cause death as a result of oxygen deficiency, and from the toxic effects of the gases themselves.[1]

The abnormal colon flora, to a lesser degree, produces the same volatile, toxic by-products that killed the farm workers. Is it any wonder many people are sick and dying before their natural time? A slow and invisible process is destroying health from the inside.

Let us take a closer look at these toxic chemicals produced in the abnormal colon flora and examine how they enter the bloodstream to affect the whole body.

A healthy bloodstream is a direct result of the normal flora in the colon. If the colon flora is abnormal, toxins are generated and circulate in the bloodstream. Colon problems are here to stay unless the cause is removed directly from the colon, where pathogens and parasites can live, multiply, and excrete toxins. The toxins we are considering here are insidious bacterial by-products that eventually weaken the immune system on the molecular level. Table 2 presents only a few of the toxins produced in the abnormal colon. Yet, when this partial list of toxins is added to the list of environmental toxins, it becomes obvious why degenerative diseases are increasing!

In 1994, many people in several states became seriously ill and a few died from consuming improperly cooked meat contaminated with *E. coli*. This created nationwide awareness of the danger of pathogenic bacteria.

Aminoethyl mercaptan	The by-product of decomposition of cysteine, a naturally occurring amino acid. Its presence exerts a very strong hypotensive effect.
Ammonia	A by-product of urea and protein decomposition, formed by certain bacterial species in the colon. Normally, ammonia is converted to urea. When this conversion fails to occur, ammonia causes neurological symptoms and may be involved with malignant transformation of cells.
Histamine	Formed from the decomposition of tryptophan, an amino acid, it can cause head congestion, headache, cardiac arrhythmia, nervous depression, lowered blood pressure, nausea, and collapse.
Hydrogen sulfide gas	A by-product of protein decomposition, this gas irritates the inner lining of the colon and can be as toxic as cyanide in comparable amounts. It can cause weakness, rapid pulse rate, nausea, and death.
Indole	A by-product of tryptophan decomposition. A diet high in meat consumption increases indole, sometimes referred to as indican. A normally functioning liver is able to detoxify indole.
Phenol or carbolic acid	A putrefactive by-product of tyrosine decomposition in the colon, causing necrosis (death of the tissues) of the gastrointestinal mucosa and liver cells.
Skatole	Another by-product of tryptophan decomposition, related to malabsorption syndrome and anemias. When in excess, skatole can circulate through the blood, resulting in foul odor emanating from the breath and stool. Skatole antagonizes acetylcholine and potassium.
Tyramine	A putrefactive by-product formed from the decomposition of the amino acid tyrosine and structurally similar to epinephrine. When it circulates in the bloodstream, it can raise blood pressure and cause central nervous system problems.

Table 2. Toxins Produced in an Unhealthy Colon[2]

When meat is cooked at sufficiently high temperatures for a proper length of time, E. *coli* is destroyed. The curious thing about E. *coli* is that many strains are considered harmless and, in fact, experts consider it to be a normal constituent of the colon flora. This microorganism, a member of the family Enterobacteriaceae, is the most commonly found bacterium in clinical specimens.[3]

E. *coli* is the largest cause of urinary tract infections.[4] It also causes diarrhea and creates an enterotoxin similar to that produced by *Vibrio cholerae*.[5] It will grow with or without oxygen and is found worldwide. As we saw in a previous chapter, research shows E. *coli's* increasing resistance to antibiotics and its ability to transmit this genetically stored resistance information across species.

Enterobacteriaceae is a large family containing other pathogenic species such as *Salmonella* and *Shigella*. Currently, *Salmonella* is frequently found in poultry products. These foods must be carefully cooked to avoid infection.

Salmonella is the most commonly reported cause of foodborne outbreaks. According to the Centers for Disease Control (CDC), about 40,000 cases of salmonellosis are reported each year. The CDC estimates that perhaps as many as 100 times more cases go unreported. This represents a twofold increase from the 1960s, when reported cases numbered 20,000. Occurrences are usually due to consuming raw or undercooked foods, especially meat, poultry, milk, or eggs.[6]

In the colon, putrefactive bacteria, which can only exist in alkaline pH, excrete gas. People frequently complain about persistent flatulence (gas), existing in the presence or absence of constipation.

While some gas may be a fermentation product of poor digestion, some is due to swallowed air. Flatulence as a result of consuming beans, raw broccoli, or wrong food combinations (such as fruit after protein or fatty foods), can usually be identified quickly because it is temporary and passes out of the colon readily.

Approximately one-third of the human population carries methane-producing members of the Archaeobacteria family in their colon, resulting in constant production of methane gas. Methane, as you recall, was one of the toxins that killed farmers in the manure pits.[7]

Some bacteria secrete such strong toxins that people get ill from them immediately. The severity of illness may range from a stomach upset to violent illness and sometimes death. These are only a few dramatic examples of how strong, aggressive bacteria can affect our health. Many more examples exist.

Breast Cancer: The Colon Flora Connection

In 1974, colon and rectal cancer accounted for an estimated 92,500 new cases in the United States. At that time, this statistic exceeded the annual rate for new cancers at any other organ site.[8] In 1993, colorectal cancer rated fourth highest in overall incidence, just after breast cancer, lung cancer, and prostate cancer. For women, colorectal cancer rated second in frequency, while for men it was third.[9]

The environment is thought to cause 80% to 90% of human cancers.[10] Over the last 20 years, medical researchers have discovered that bacteria play a key role in many diseases, among them cancer. The abnormal colon flora has been found to be directly linked to the formation of some human cancers. Bacteria in the colon modify substances they come in contact with and influence the human internal environment.[11] Data suggests a correlation between a higher fecal pH (an alkaline pH), the composition of the colon microflora, and an increased risk of colon cancer.[12,13]

Around the turn of the last century, the fathers of contemporary medicine at the Pasteur Institute in Paris established that as flowing water eventually reaches the lowest level on land, molecular toxins in the bloodstream flow to the weakest area in the system. Once toxic accumulation challenges a weak area, such as fatty breast tissue, tumors or cancer can result.[14] Everything is cause and effect.

Many bacteria are found to be capable of modifying a "wide range of environmental chemicals and in particular intestinal bacteria can modify food additives..., digestive secretions like bile salts and hormones..."[15]

Strong evidence points to a connection between both breast and colon cancer and colon bacteria.[16,17,18,19,20] Studies show *E. coli* can synthesize a known carcinogen, ethionine.[21] *Clostridium paraputrificum* may be implicated in transforming bile acids into potential carcinogens.[22] Estrogens stimulate tumor growth, and some experts state certain forms of estrogens actually may be a cause of tumors. What is not widely known, however, is that colon bacteria in the abnormal flora can apparently produce estrogens and other carcinogens from biliary steroids and bile acids present in the colon.[23,24,25,26]

High-fat diets tend to increase the amount of biliary steroids found in the colon. The colon flora of people who eat high-fat diets contains a higher percentage of types of bacteria that can produce estrone and estradiol forms of estrogen, which are linked with tumor growth.[27]

There are several types of estrogens occurring naturally in the body. Of the three most important types of estrogen (estrone, estradiol, and estriol), estradiol is found to be the most stimulating to the breast. In fact, it is 1,000 times more stimulating to the breast than estriol. Estradiol is also found to increase one's risk of breast cancer.[28]

Some bile acids have been shown to be carcinogenic, while others can be converted by bacterial action into potent carcinogens.[29] In 1994, a study found bile acids in breast cyst fluid that were proven to be of intestinal origin.[30]

The highest incidence of breast and colon cancers is found in developed nations, where diets are highest in fat and animal protein and lowest in cereal fibers.[31,32,33,34] Dietary factors have a great influence on the colon flora.[35,36,37,38]

Thus, diet can promote either health or disease, not only through nutrition, but also by affecting the colon flora. The type of bacteria contained in the colon chamber has a profound impact on the level of our health. Some studies now conclude that low fecal pH is more relevant in decreasing the incidence of colon cancer than the role of dietary fiber.[39]

Balance Lost

When toxins overwhelm the body, balance is lost. We are not naturally sick. We become imbalanced, then we become sick. Illness is an end result. Imbalance originates in the colon; thus, balance must be reestablished in the colon flora.

This chapter has presented striking examples of the role of our colon microflora on our health. Once disease has progressed to the extreme point of a cancer, adjusting the colon pH is not sufficient to effect a change in a process already deeply rooted in the system.

Understanding and applying research can help us prevent such extremes in the future. By promoting a healthy colon flora, the colon can be maintained at a slightly acidic pH. Thus we can increase our resistance to disease, our enjoyment of good health and an extended life.

CHAPTER 9

Autointoxication Explained

Two words, "toxin" and "autointoxication," embrace key principles to understanding the deleterious effect an unbalanced colon flora has upon human health.

What exactly is a toxin? It is generally recognized to mean any poisonous substance. *The New Shorter Oxford English Dictionary* defines a toxin as, "Any poisonous antigenic substance produced by or derived from micro-organisms, which causes disease when present at low concentration in the body."[1] According to *Taber's Cyclopedic Medical Dictionary*, toxin can be more briefly defined as, "A poisonous substance of animal or plant origin."[2] Toxins are not the pathogens themselves, but are substances produced by the pathogens.

Autointoxication is defined as a condition that results when poisonous substances are produced within the body.[3] Although not recognized officially by modern medicine, autointoxication is the predecessor to many diseases. This process can take place in our bodies, and we will explore some of the routes by which this happens.

Where do toxins come from? Previous chapters have clearly shown us what happens when pathogens gain hold in an unhealthy colon. The secretions of these pathogenic microorganisms, whether bacteria, parasites, or other organisms, are toxins that cause varying amounts of damage to the host. These toxins can migrate to other sites in the body, causing autointoxication and, eventually, disease.

Factors determining the site, type, and degree of disease include the type of pathogen, strength of its toxins, number of pathogens present, the resistance or immunity of the host, and the areas of the host's body already in a weakened state.

Some pathogens are extremely virulent and can cause severe illness and death quite quickly. Others, such as *Candida albicans* and most parasites, are more insidious in nature. They can even exist for many years in a healthy person and take over when trauma or illness results in a weakened immune system. They can be present unnoticed for a long time, showing no visible effects until the balance is tipped in their favor.

Vegetarians and the Toxic Colon

Many vegetarians believe they are free of toxins because they eat no meat and have a good diet. This is all relative. A healthy diet alone will not correct an unhealthy colon flora. It is like strewing the best quality of seeds on the poorest of soils. Nothing will happen. Many vegetarians have toxic colons.

Amino acids, the basic components of protein, are found in all cells of living tissue and form the building blocks of all cells in our body. Even vegetarians have protein substances arriving in their colon, which can cause problems when the colon flora is already unbalanced. This is illustrated in the following story told by Dr. Empringham.

Substitute the words "protein" or "amino acids" where he dramatically says "meat," and the picture becomes clearer.

"What is the matter with me?" said a patient the other day. "I have been ailing a long time, but no one seems able to find out what is wrong."

"Your trouble comes from meat," I remarked. "The analysis we have made proves that poisons are continually seeping into your blood from dead flesh decomposing in your colon."

The man laughed and said, "Meat! You think my troubles are caused by meat! Why, I have not eaten a morsel of meat for 30 years — nothing but fruits and vegetables."

I said, "Yes, I know. You gave this information to the physician who took your history the day you came to see us. Nevertheless, your excreta contains meat. This would not matter, but unfortunately, your colon is cursed with putrefactive bacteria generating virulent toxins from your refuse."

Of course, there is nothing unusual about the colon residues containing meat. That is true of every human being, including those who live exclusively on fruits and vegetables. Even excreta from sheep, cows, and rabbits that eat nothing but grass, contain meat. This is because the body of every creature consists of billions of microscopic cells, and every minute some of these die and are swept into the colon... These dead cells are perfectly harmless if they do not come in contact with putrefactive bacteria.[4]

Autointoxication

There are two main sources of toxins emanating from the colon. The first source is from the by-products of an unhealthy colon flora. A second source is the result of improper functioning of the ileocecal valve.

The ileocecal valve is located between the end of the small intestine and the beginning of the large intestine. It is a doorway that opens into the cecum at the lower part of the ascending colon. The valve opens only in one direction, preventing waste material from reentering the small intestine. In some people, the valve does not shut completely. In these cases, bacteria can be forced into the lower small intestine, the ileum, where food absorption is still taking place.[5] The presence of fecal material and bacteria in the ileum can contaminate the lymphatic system and bloodstream, as material from the ileum passes directly into these areas.

Just how do toxins manufactured in the colon affect the rest of the body? Toxins are transported, as a matter of course, from the colon through the portal vein to the liver. To understand how this happens, a short lesson in blood circulation is helpful.

Blood circulates through the body in two kinds of blood vessels. The arteries carry fresh, oxygenated blood (red blood) from the heart to supply all the organs and tissues of the body. The veins carry waste materials away from the organs and tissues. Venous blood does not contain oxygen (it is blue) and returns to the heart. From the heart, blood passes to the lungs to become re-oxygenated, becoming red blood again. It then reenters the heart before circulating once more through the arteries.

Names for arteries and veins correspond to the part of the body being supplied with blood. In the abdominal region, the superior and inferior mesenteric arteries are the major arteries that carry fresh blood to the colon. Likewise, mesenteric veins carry blood and other substances away from the colon.

The inferior mesenteric vein carries blood away from the rectum and sigmoid and descending colon. The superior mesenteric veins return blood from the small intestine, the cecum, and from the ascending and transverse portions of the colon. The inferior mesenteric vein empties into the splenic vein, which comes from the spleen. The splenic vein and superior mesenteric veins join to form the portal vein. The portal vein lies about level with the second lumbar vertebra and passes upward into the liver.

The liver is made up of tiny units called "lobules." Each lobule is composed of cells that are closely interspersed with many blood vessels. Blood from the portal vein reaches each of these lobules through smaller veins and capillaries. From here, the blood returns to the inferior vena cava, located on the back of the liver, which carries the deoxygenated blood up to the heart.

The liver has a multitude of functions. It processes nutrients, including carbohydrates, fats, and proteins, carried to it through the venous circulation. As the main organ of detoxification in the body, the liver protects the body from harmful substances. It breaks toxins down and transforms them into harmless compounds that can be excreted from the body.

Macrophages, found throughout the body, are one of the most important cell types actively involved in the immune response. Macrophages specifically defend against microorganisms and harmful chemicals.

Some macrophages wander about certain areas of the body. Others remain fixed in specific locations. Large quantities exist in the spleen, lymph nodes, alveoli, and tonsils. About 50% of all macro-

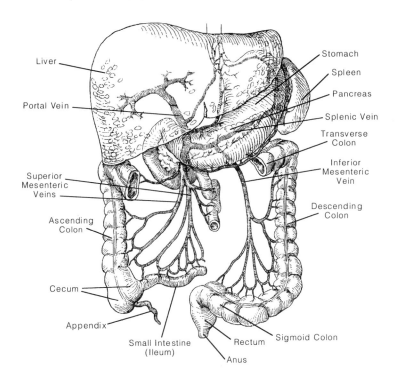

Figure 5. Portal Vein System

phages are concentrated in the liver, where they are called "Kupffer cells." Kupffer cells are embedded in the lining of the sinusoids of the liver and constitute a large percentage of liver cells. Kupffer cells have phagocytic activity and protect the body from microorganisms that may have entered the portal system from the colon.[6,7,8,9]

The liver is constantly accumulating and distributing blood. It circulates about 1.5 liters of blood per minute, and 70% of this blood flow arrives from the portal vein.[10] Waste products and toxins from the colon that are not properly detoxified by the liver can go on to affect all tissues of the body.

Even basic anatomy books state that both nutrients and waste materials are carried into the liver from the portal vein along with various "...toxic substances harmful to the tissues of the body."[11] Thus, it can clearly be seen how the colon affects the condition of the blood.

Even in seemingly healthy people, hundreds of substances originating from the colon can escape across the colon's mucosal border. All of these need to be detoxified by the liver, presuming it is not already overloaded.[12]

The colon and the liver are analogous to the oil pan and the oil filter in an automobile motor. As in auto maintenance, we must ensure that the filter is clean at all times in order to preserve the life of the motor. To purge the liver while allowing the colon to continue polluting the bloodstream is like replacing the oil filter and not changing the oil.

The colon is currently the main source of pollution in our system. This is not the function nature intended. If intestinal putrefaction is excessive or if the liver cells have been challenged or fail to function, toxic by-products enter general circulation and produce the condition known as autointoxication.

Allergies and Colon Flora

The toxins emanating from the abnormal colon flora appear to be directly related to food allergies. Allergies are widespread. They can be caused by genetics, environmental or chemical factors, and foods. Allergies are generally recognized as the system reacting inappropriately to certain foods or other substances.

I have seen food allergies reduced in about 50% of people after their system eliminated the accumulated fecal material and a firm foundation of healthy colon flora was reestablished.

There are many theories in holistic medicine relating allergies to a polluted bloodstream. If this is the case, then the colon must be addressed initially as a prime source of internal pollution.

Autointoxication, the Colon and Indican

Since blood circulation is constant, the liver does its best to detoxify anything coming into it from the colon. When the liver is overworked because the colon is abnormal, it is challenged beyond its capacity, the bloodstream is polluted, and internal infections are possible.

Next in line, the kidneys become challenged, and toxins move into the bladder. Puffiness under the eyes is often the first indication that the kidneys are being challenged.[13]

The bladder, in an attempt to remove the onslaught of toxic waste, may wake us up at night to urinate even when fluids were not taken before retiring. The inherent wisdom of the body struggles to cleanse itself and stay alive.

Dr. Empringham spoke of indican as an indicator of toxicity in the colon. Although this urine test is rarely used today, medical professionals may want to consider reevaluating its validity. I offer the following story, written in 1940, letting Dr. Empringham speak from his own experience as a microbiologist.

> The difference between the old and new methods of urinalysis is very great. For example, in [America] little importance is paid to indican. This toxin comes from residues decomposing in the bowels. It is found in the urine of almost every civilized person. Therefore, formerly, doctors thought indican natural. In America most laboratory reports say, "Indican - Normal." But we now know this poison is *never normal.* It is usual but not normal, natural, or necessary.[14]

Empringham states that when the native flora is restored to the colon, a person's urinalysis will show no trace of indican.

Unseen Health Problems

Many individuals appear healthy and have a good appetite, no aches or pains. Nothing suggests a problem in their colon, and yet a good stool test may show an alkaline pH that is producing pathogens and yeasts in abundance. Why is this?

In establishing the strength of bridges and buildings, architects provide a large margin of safety. Likewise, important organs such as the lungs, kidneys, and adrenal glands are in pairs. Each one of the pair is more than capable of doing all the work required of the two in health. The same principle of tremendous reserve power is true of

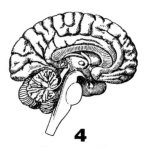

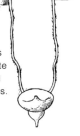

5

The kidney and urinary bladder are also overwhelmed by excess toxins. This can contribute to kidney problems and chronic bladder infections.

4

Toxins can affect the brain and nervous system, causing headaches and other symptoms. Some toxins can cross the blood-brain barrier.

3

Toxins leave the liver and enter the bloodstream. They flow through the body, affecting the weakest body areas.

2

Toxins are not completely broken down by the already challenged liver.

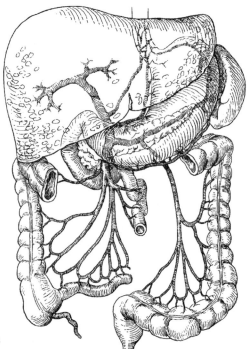

1

Alkaline colon pH. Toxins formed in the colon flow through the mesenteric veins, into the portal vein, and then into the liver.

Figure 6. Unhealthy Colon Function

1

Predominance and maintenance of healthy colon flora with a slightly acidic pH ensures an insignificant amount of toxins are formed in the colon. Portal system transport from colon to liver consists mainly of nutrients formed by the lactobacteria flora.

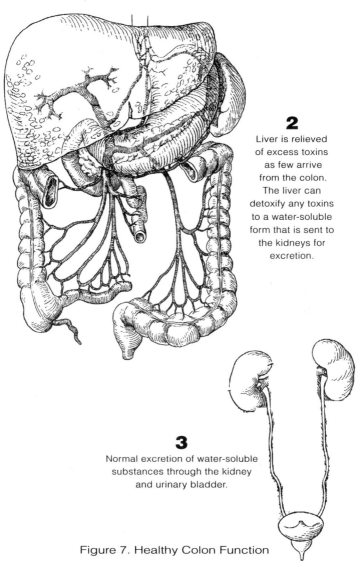

2

Liver is relieved of excess toxins as few arrive from the colon. The liver can detoxify any toxins to a water-soluble form that is sent to the kidneys for excretion.

3

Normal excretion of water-soluble substances through the kidney and urinary bladder.

Figure 7. Healthy Colon Function

the organs that are not in pairs, such as the heart, liver, and skin.

For years after a portion of their stomach was removed, some people have lived in good health because their small intestine had enough reserve power to perform. This reserve is responsible for the sense of good health many people feel. However, this sense of health continues only as long as the body possesses a surplus of protective power.

When this reserve declines or when the immune system is weakened, toxins will affect the weakest part of the body. It is only when the weakness has become pronounced and the toxins strong enough to do some real damage, that disease will be diagnosed. True prevention means building a good foundation of health and maintaining an abundant reserve of health.

CHAPTER 10

Aging and Mental Health: The Colon Connection

Let us again use the analogy of the automobile and the human body. Race cars maintained in excellent condition can run smoothly for years and achieve speeds of 200 miles per hour. Why? Because they are balanced and clean inside. The oil that goes up into the motor and circulates through the oil filter is not challenged with dirty oil. The exhaust is not impacted with waste, the cars are immaculately maintained, inside and out.

All that moves, from the microcosm to the macrocosm, man to machine, share processes of intake or ingestion, combustion or digestion, exhaust or elimination. In all human or mechanical processes, cleanliness facilitates correct function.

Disease can only exist in a proper medium. A healthy soil grows a healthy plant. By changing the medium to normal, starting from the foundation up, there should be no disease. This foundation is the colon.

Time Does Not Make Us Old

Dr. Empringham suggests we should live much longer than we do and explains why we do not. The average life span of civilized human beings is shorter than nature intended, and science may someday enable humanity to maintain youthfulness for a much longer period.

While at the University of Odessa, Eli Metchnikoff became a student and follower of Owen, a comparative anatomist. Owen found the colons of many adults to be filled with trillions of harmful, putrefactive bacteria, generating toxic by-products. He did not find this condition in healthy animals. Owen attributed the failure of humans to live to a ripe old age to his finding of intestinal toxemia.

Apparently, this was a clue that Metchnikoff followed in his studies, for he became fascinated with prolonging the human life span and did extensive research on colon health. One of Metchnikoff's favored theories described the relationship of poisons excreted by certain bacterial species in the colon to senility.[1]

A glance through the microscope proves that the body of every living being is merely an assemblage of tiny cells. Each one of these cells is a complete entity that breathes, eats, drinks, and excretes waste. At the end of a few weeks, which is its life span, the cell dies.

Each of these microscopic living cells which compose our bodies gives birth to a successor before it expires. Therefore, our bodies are in continual flux. Little by little, every day we die; just as gradually and continuously, every moment, cell by cell, we are being reborn.

What is the cause of those changes we attribute to age? What is the cause of the phenomenon we call "natural death"? This is one of the most profound questions of biology. The answer is that, before our cells generate successors, they are continually poisoned and sometimes destroyed by unchecked toxins circulating in the bloodstream. Although this destruction of cells is a natural process, it is too often accelerated in modern society.

Sometimes the cells are replaced by dead matter instead of by new cells. This is what is known as "arteriosclerosis," or "hardening of the arteries." Our blood vessels lose their natural elasticity as cells are replaced with inorganic mineral salts, fat, or other materials. As a result of this accumulation inside the vessels, the blood vessel's diameter decreases. Because of this smaller passageway, more effort by the heart is required to maintain circulation. While these are spoken of as "normal" symptoms of increasing age, in reality, the number of years we have lived has nothing to do with such degenerative changes due to an unhealthy lifestyle and diet. The toxins from the resulting unhealthy colon stress an already overburdened liver, spill into the bloodstream, and affect other areas of the body.

Many people are not tired from overwork but rather think they are overworked because the labor they previously enjoyed has now become fatiguing. This is a condition of toxic fatigue. Normal fatigue is quickly cured by rest, but resting will not relieve a toxic condition. If one feels tired when arising after eight hours of sleep, the cause can be found in the toxins retained during sleep in the liver, heart, kidneys, and colon.

During breastfeeding, the infant's colon is completely covered with *B. bifidum*, a single-celled, protective, beneficial bacterium that produces acids. *B. bifidum* is often compared to white corpuscles that defend the bloodstream, but these two are entirely different and protect us in different ways. White corpuscles destroy bacteria by devouring them. Lactobacteria in the colon generate mild acids that are fatal or extremely injurious to all putrefactive, poisonous types of bacteria. Unfortunately, the majority of people have entirely lost this protective flora because, in ignorance, it was not maintained from birth.

Putrefactive bacteria, multiplying in the colon, generate toxins that leak into the system through absorption. Gradually over time, every gland, organ, and cellular tissue of the human body is injured. This is the cause of most changes we falsely attribute to aging. These toxins eventually bring on almost every kind of degenerative disease, cutting our natural lifetime approximately in half![2,3]

Mind, Emotion, Body

The inability to function well in society is not a new manifestation. In 1929, N.W. Kaiser, M.D., reported his studies concerning the relationship between colon hygiene and mental disorders. In his report, he cited many other doctors who contributed to this field of research.

Dr. Kaiser considered constipation to be a probable cause of many obscure psychoses and to be responsible for such symptoms as apathy, irritability, melancholia, mania and, in some extreme cases, even suicidal inclinations.[4]

The following study is from an actual test of mental patients with constipation at Toledo State Hospital, Ohio in 1930.[5] The purpose of testing was to determine if constipation was the causative factor in mental problems or if mental problems were the cause of constipation.

In this study, constipation was defined as relative to the time required to eliminate barium meal. According to most medical authorities, the normal time to eliminate barium meal taken orally is between 36 and 48 hours. When elimination from the colon exceeds 48 hours, it is considered constipation.

Eighty percent of the 70 patients tested required more than 48 hours to eliminate the barium meal from their colon. One female manic-depressive patient required an amazing 240 hours before the barium meal was entirely eliminated.

These patients were given several colon hygiene water treatments. The mental conditions of many patients improved so greatly that they were released from the mental hospital. However, some of these patients returned due to recurrence.

This demonstrates the limitations of plain water colonics. They will clear impactions but are not effective to prevent relapse. It does not matter how many colon treatments are given if replacement of the normal colon flora is left out of the clinical treatment.

Dr. Kaiser's ideas were scoffed at by others and, as a result, his work went largely ignored for decades. If we consider the connections between the unhealthy colon flora, an alkaline colon, and the toxins that circulate as a result of constipation, Dr. Kaiser's ideas do not seem at all ridiculous.

In health, the colon is acidic and fermentation is in control, existing as the result of a normal flora. In the case of delayed bowel movements or alteration of the normal flora, putrefactive organisms become predominant. The colon contents become alkaline and toxins are generated.

Where constipation has persisted for long periods, the tissues become saturated with toxins, impairing the liver and kidneys to the extent that degenerative structural and functional changes can occur. Many toxins created in the putrefactive colon are capable of crossing the blood-brain barrier and have known mental effects. Examples of these are found in Chapter 8, Table 2, *Toxins Produced in an Unhealthy Colon.*

Histamine can cause nervous depression, tyramine can cause central nervous system problems. Skatole antagonizes acetylcholine, which is important in brain function and nerve signal transmission. The total effects of toxins crossing the blood-brain barrier are so great that it is impossible to recognize a complete class of symptoms. They can include anorexia, flatulence, constipation, nausea, bad breath, or diarrhea.

No one can predict when actual illness will appear. Some early symptoms include backache, headache, aching joints, neuralgia, neuritis, and attacks of asthma. The onset of physical symptoms is gradual at first but, unless resolved, may progress into mental symptoms such as lassitude, depression, fatigue, sleeplessness, lack of concentration, and loss of memory.[6] As time goes on, more serious problems can arise.

In 1932, Dr. Schellberg stated the medical profession was beginning to appreciate the importance of constipation in the mentally disturbed. Nervous impulses from the abdominal cavity passing to the brain through the vagus and sympathetic nerve pathways were reported to directly affect the sense of well-being and give rise to acute mental distress. These symptoms and conditions were lessened by removing the pathogenic condition in the colon.[7]

Harvey Kellogg, M.D. suggested most civilized people were suffering from constipation and intestinal toxemia.[8] In the United States, kidney disease has occurred only since about 1900, which has been attributed by some to the wearing down of the immune system. Dr. Kellogg linked kidney disease to the tremendous toxic overload the system has had to deal with in the air and food, which ends up in the colon and then finds its way into the bloodstream.

In 1930, the Royal Society of Medicine of Great Britain held a meeting on intestinal toxemia. Sixty leading physicians attended. It was reported that constipation caused accentuated mental symptoms such as melancholia, irritability, mania, and suicidal tendencies. Physically, a long string of degenerative diseases was also reported as arising from constipation.[9]

Why was this initial research discontinued when it showed a possible cause to a major worldwide health problem? Currently, a few researchers are rediscovering the colon connection. A recent article by Jeffrey Bland, Ph.D. in chemistry, stated there are possible links (in combination with other factors) between colon-produced pathogens, the liver's detoxifying ability, and Parkinson's disease, Alzheimer's, and even schizophrenia.[10]

When the liver, the primary organ of detoxification in the body, is overwhelmed, toxins circulate in the body. A study of brain-injured children in Philadelphia, Pennsylvania found many of them to have impaired colon and liver function. A direct connection was made between toxins originating in the colon that overloaded the liver and had an adverse effect on brain chemistry.[11]

Another finding relates to benzodiazepine, the active ingredient in the pharmaceutical drug most commonly known by the trade name "Valium." Several researchers have found high levels of a benzodiazepine-like substance in the bloodstreams of certain individuals. The levels were high enough to alter brain chemistry. However, none of the patients had ever taken benzodiazepine-based drugs. There are currently two theories as to the possible origin of this substance in their blood: synthesis from bacteria in the colon or production from nitrogenous compounds in the liver.[12]

In the first half of this book, we have explored modern scientific evidence showing that, in fact, much disease originates in the colon. The examples included diseases attributed to old age and mental disturbances.

For many reasons, such as antibiotic overuse and diet, our protective colon flora has been partially or completely destroyed. This leaves the colon open for habitation by pathogenic bacteria, yeasts, and parasites. Toxins produced by these microorganisms create a polluted colon and can directly influence other tissues and organs of our body. This is the condition known as "autointoxication."

The weakest areas of the body are affected first and foremost. These weaknesses may be inherited or acquired during the wear and tear of life. After the passage of time, other sites may become affected as well. Depending on the type of damage that has occurred and its location, modern medicine can offer a diagnosis, labeling the disease process that has now set in.

The essential area that must be addressed in most cases is the colon flora, which is the foundation of the body. Many researchers throughout history have studied and worked with the colon as a means to attain both health and longevity.

Let us now take a look at the vast history of medical, scientific, and microbiological work in this area.

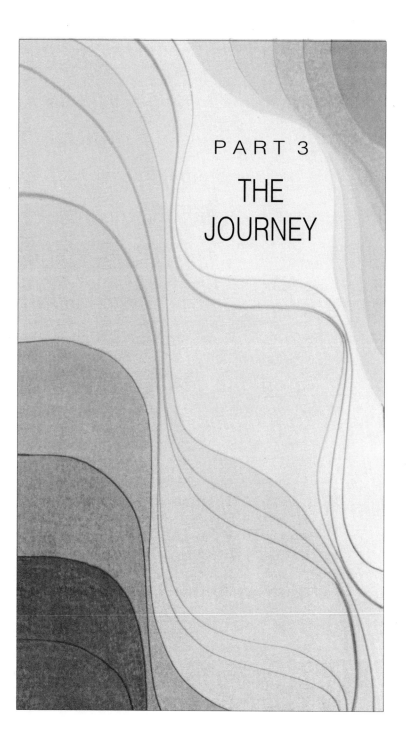

PART 3

THE
JOURNEY

CHAPTER 11

Colon in the Quest for Health

Throughout history, the colon has played an important role in the quest for health. Around the globe, the colon's role in disease was recognized and addressed. All cultures, since the beginning of recorded history, included specific methods for cleansing the colon in their health care. Only in modern times have these practices fallen by the wayside, the knowledge shelved as other issues in modern medicine have taken precedence.

To bring the ancient art of colon therapy into the 21st century, many old myths must be dispelled, and information with procedures based on scientific principles must be introduced. To accomplish this, it is helpful to understand some pertinent ancient and modern history.

In this section of the book, we will explore the rich history and legacy of colon health. When we arrive at the present, we will explore what is going on today in this field. Then, we will see where this research can take us in the future and discover the future has already arrived.

Ancient Use of Enemas

The use of enemas is documented from 5,000 years ago through the present time. Humans have always instinctively felt the colon was a source of disease. Ancient practitioners used a variety of methods to cleanse the colon. Usually, it was by means of the enema, which is still used today. Many varieties of enemas have existed, and enema methodology has continued to evolve over the centuries.

Cleansing of the colon using enemas has been recorded since ancient times in Egypt, Babylonia, Assyria, Greece, Italy, Germany, Holland, France, Arabia, Africa, Hawaii, India, and China. This procedure was considered important for physical health.

Evidence shows enemas may have been used during the dynasty of the pharaohs in Egypt. Egyptian legend says this practice was derived from observation of the ibis, a bird similar to the stork. Ancient Egyptians noticed the ibis seemed to use its beak to inject water into its anus. Whether or not this was what the bird was actually doing, the legend persisted.[1]

Enemas were also utilized by some societies as part of their spiritual practice or spiritual purification. An Arabic text found in the Vatican and Hapsburg libraries, translated by Dr. Edmond Szekely, mentions that Christ required his disciples to fast for seven days and to take enemas prior to joining him. In these writings, Christ is said to have suggested that the diet of his church be lactovegetarian (meaning a vegetarian diet that includes dairy products). Other faiths, such as the Jewish, Shiite Moslem, Hindu, and Essene religions, also required cleansing of the colon.[2]

Hippocrates, who is called the "Father of Medicine," used both enemas and suppositories containing various ingredients. He recommended enemas primarily for those with a robust constitution who were not eliminating properly; he recommended suppositories for those with a weak constitution. Other ancient Greek physicians, such as Galen in the second century AD, utilized enemas in their practice as well.

Chang Chung Ching, whom some call the "Chinese Hippocrates," used enemas and allegedly preferred them to cathartic herbs.[3] Cathartic herbs are those that strongly purge the bowels and usually have an irritating effect on the colon's walls.

Ayurvedic medicine, from India, dates back as far as 5,000 years and is practiced in America today. Ayurveda utilizes a variety of enemas and colon cleanses administered according to body type, constitution, and disease syndrome.[4] Based on these criteria, many different substances were used in Ayurvedic enemas. For example, sesame oil was thought to provide lubrication to the colon wall. However, these substances have no lasting effect in normalizing the colon flora or restoring the slightly acidic pH.

Avicenna was a renowned Arabian physician who lived from 980 AD to 1036 AD. Like the Ayurveds of India, Avicenna also recommended oil enemas for the elderly, who tend to have constipation due to dryness. He wrote:

> The enema is an excellent agent for getting rid of the superfluities of the intestinal tract as well as for allaying pains over the kidneys and bladder and for relieving inflammatory conditions of these organs and also for relieving pain and for drawing superfluities from the vital organs of the upper parts of the body.[5]

Enemas were known in the Americas as well. Native American medicine men included the enema as part of treatment. Prior to Spanish occupation, the great Mayan culture in Central America is documented to have used enemas, as did the Aztecs for general listlessness and pains due to colon problems.[6] The health practices of Mexican cultures also included the use of enemas.[7]

The enema's history, of course, includes the development of tools used to administer it. Throughout the world, all kinds of instruments were made from gourds, reeds, animal horns, animal skin or bladders to form what we know in modern times as the enema bag or syringe. In Polynesia, Hawaiian kahunas (who were both medical practitioners and spiritual leaders) used gourds to administer their enemas and empty the colon. The enemas usually contained herbal ingredients infused in water.

Gourds were also used in other areas of the world. In certain African tribes, a hollow cow horn was used.[8] Other cultures made various instruments such as syringes from natural materials.

Western World

In European countries, enemas were utilized by many practitioners, both famous and unknown. These practitioners made valuable contributions to the technique and developed new tools for administering the enema.

Regnier de Graaf was a prominent Dutch physician who lived from 1641 to 1673. He studied medicine in Holland, England, and France, specializing in research and anatomical study. He was the first to study pancreatic function and secretions and to recognize the importance of pancreatic juice in digestion. In 1672, he was also the first to describe the structure of what we now call the Graafian follicles in the ovaries.

In his medical practice, de Graaf used enemas and even created a syringe that patients could use at home for their ease and convenience. Up until this time, assistance was necessary for administration of enemas. This invention took considerable time and experimentation. He also wrote a major work that contained much information about proper use of the enema, including when it should be administered and contraindications.[9]

He classified enemas according to the actions of their contents. These classifications included "emollient," "purgative," "astringent," and "nutrient" categories. However, de Graaf established the fact that use of highly medicated enemas did not produce clear results. He himself

> ...preferred the simple pure water enema or sea water to which there had been an addition of a small amount of salt or urine of a normal individual if the condition of the patient warranted more active treatment. ...These liquids have the power to dissolve hardened material in the bowel and at the same time stimulate the organ and cause expulsion of the dissolved matter. They therefore fulfill a double purpose.[10]

Dr. de Graaf was almost on the right track, and made many very important advancements. He recommended the enema for intestinal ailments such as colic, diarrhea, and worms. He also found it effective for problems in the bladder, kidney, and uterus, and for relief of headaches. Like the Chinese physician Chang Chung Ching, de Graaf found enemas far preferable to using purgative substances, which are very strong and irritating to the system, especially for very ill or weak patients.[11]

Freidrich Hoffmann of Halle, a highly respected physician of his time, recommended enemas in the first half of the 18th century. His book, *Practice of Medicine*, included information on administration of enemas and was translated from Latin into English in 1783.[12]

In 1790, Frederick Hildebrandt, professor at Braunschweig, authored three volumes on the history of impurities in the stomach and intestines. In his work, he noted the value of enemas when used appropriately and observed the poor results due to misuse of the procedure.[13]

In the early 1800s, more improvements were made on enema apparatus, and doctors continued to utilize the method and write about the technique and its usefulness. European and American physicians incorporated enemas into their practice.

Until the 20th century, extreme measures were used to cleanse the colon. These included herbal remedies, oils, medications, and even tobacco smoke blown into the colon.[14] Some of these procedures were harmful, while others had no lasting results. The enema, nonetheless, represents the first attempt at normalizing the colon.

The apparatus used ranged from natural objects to professional tools. However, medicine was about to develop a practitioner-assisted apparatus and methodology. With the advances made in science, microbiologists would soon shed much light on exactly how to promote true colon health by restoring the natural colon ecology.

CHAPTER 12

The Fathers of Colon Microbiology

Scientists have been on an extended quest, seeking ways to prolong life and strengthen the immune system. This quest has led them to investigate how the body is able to function and respond to the world around it.

Without the microscope, there would be no medical science as we know it today. The microscope has allowed us to see and discover new worlds of life and knowledge. With the electron microscope, scientists can perceive minute life-forms such as viruses, allowing the science of microbiology to develop to where it is today.

This book is based on a lineage of scientific research. At the core of this lineage are two master microbiologists, Eli Metchnikoff and James Empringham. The quest of these two men led them to answers that can assist medicine today. Researchers around the world are quietly continuing their work. In research articles, authors repeatedly refer back to Metchnikoff and his original work. However, until now, this research has lain on library shelves gathering dust. Only now, through my work, is this knowledge being clinically applied. Only now is it reaching the general public.

Louis Pasteur

The knowledge of the colon's significance to overall health has its foundation in the sciences of microbiology and chemistry. These disciplines form the core of information for health professionals worldwide. This core knowledge began with the work of Louis Pasteur, a French chemist who lived from 1822 to 1895. He established the Pasteur Institute in 1888.

Louis Pasteur divided bacteria into two main classes: (1) the pathogens, which are disease-producing organisms, and (2) the saprophytes, which live only on dead, decaying organic matter.[1] Saprophyte spores are abundant on meat, often survive cooking, and cause food to spoil. These putrefactive bacteria cannot function in the normal colon, which has a slightly acid pH. Although Pasteur considered these saprophytes harmless, his associate, Eli Metchnikoff, was to prove him wrong.

Pasteur considered bacteria to be the causative agents of disease. He stated that, first and foremost, bacteria must be combated in order to treat disease. Pasteur's germ theory is the basis for the medical model of the fight against germs.

Pierre Jacque Antoine Bechamp

Pierre Bechamp was a physician, chemist, naturalist, and biochemist. A contemporary of Pasteur's, he took quite a different approach. Bechamp theorized that pathogenic bacteria will only establish themselves on already diseased or decaying material. He stated that the medium was the most significant factor in determining the action of bacteria. When the body was healthy, the bacteria would be beneficial, aiding the host. When the body was in an unhealthy state, bacteria could become harmful.[2]

Evidence for Bechamp's hypothesis is found in the colon, where if the medium is correct, the beneficial bacteria grow and the pathogenic bacteria are unable to take hold. This is certainly the case with some bacteria we have seen, such as *E. coli*, which is sometimes benign and occasionally fatal. *Candida albicans* is also benign when outnumbered in the normal colon flora but, in an unhealthy colon, it overgrows and becomes a major health problem.

On his deathbed, Louis Pasteur acknowledged that Bechamp's theory was, in fact, more accurate and complete than his own.[3] Today, Bechamp's outlook is proving to be on the cutting edge of science. Modern medicine based itself on the work of Pasteur, directing its medicine primarily to killing pathogens, while doing nothing to address the basic health and medium of the body. Since this attack plan of heroic medicine has failed dramatically, science must be willing to step to a new level of understanding, as Pasteur himself was finally able to do.

In Europe today, a large number of physicians are utilizing Bechamp's paradigm as the basis for a new, well-developed approach to medicine. This work is just starting to become known in the United States.

Eli Metchnikoff

Eli Metchnikoff was the true father of research on lactobacteria and colon health. He was born on May 3, 1845, in a Russian village near Kharkow. As a young boy, he was very interested in natural history, botany, and geology and gave lectures on these topics to his peers. At the University of Kharkow, he completed a four-year course of study in only two years and pursued further studies at other universities.

In 1870, he was appointed Titular Professor of zoology and comparative anatomy at the University of Odessa, Russia, where he taught for 12 years. Between 1866 and 1892, he published several papers and texts on the topics of comparative pathology and inflammation.

Resigning from his work at the University of Odessa in 1882, Metchnikoff turned to private research and traveled extensively. He eventually moved to Paris, joining the Pasteur Institute, which was then in its second year. Metchnikoff worked with Pasteur until Pasteur's death in 1895, when he succeeded Pasteur as director of the institute.

In 1908, Eli Metchnikoff and Paul Erlich (a German bacteriologist) were awarded the Nobel prize in "Physiology or Medicine." [4] Metchnikoff was an honorary Doctor of Science at the University of Cambridge, England and was affiliated with other prominent medical societies throughout Europe.

Metchnikoff's research indicated that many degenerative organ diseases have their origin in the colon, due to putrefactive material that is not eliminated. The putrefactive bacteria multiply in the alkaline pH of the abnormal colon flora, continually spreading their toxins throughout the colon. As part of his research, Metchnikoff did extensive fecal analysis on samples from patients all over France.

Collaborating physicians supplied Metchnikoff with a patient history along with each sample. From his studies, Metchnikoff formulated the following tenets, which are still relevant today.

(1) There is a close correlation between a person's health and the type of bacteria that reside and predominate in his or her colon.

(2) When lactobacteria are absent, putrefactive bacteria dominate the colon. These bacteria decompose food, form protein residues, and generate toxins.

(3) The formation of toxins can continue for many years before there is noticeable damage to the individual's health.

(4) Since toxins generated in the colon pollute the bloodstream, the entire system is polluted. However, this pollution does not result in the same illness in each affected individual. Each person will experience the result of toxic pollution in the part of his or her body that is congenitally vulnerable. Some individuals will experience kidney disease, while others may experience damage to the pancreas, stomach ulcers, high blood pressure, or other illnesses.[5]

Eli Metchnikoff was the first person known to attempt implanting lactobacteria into the human colon. He tried both rectal and oral routes of implantation and was unsuccessful. Although his plan was effective in the test tube, it failed in the colon for multiple reasons. The strain of *Lactobacilli* he used was *Lactobacillus bulgaricus*, a bovine strain that will not implant in humans. Only a human strain of *Lactobacilli* will implant in the human colon.

Another reason these experiments succeeded in the test tube but failed in patients was that the cultures were administered orally and destroyed by the pH of the stomach acids. Therefore, the cultures did not reach the colon in a viable form.[6]

Metchnikoff, however, knew his basic theory was correct. For good health, the colon should be colonized primarily by lactobacteria. His work has inspired succeeding generations of microbiologists and researchers.

James Empringham

At the turn of this century, Dr. James Empringham was a student of Eli Metchnikoff. By the time Empringham's abilities as a scientist and physician matured, his credentials were no less than astonishing. He is truly the unsung hero of microbiology.

Empringham was Doctor of Science, Regius Professor of Microbiology at St. Margaret's in London. At one time, he served as the director of Kensington Laboratories for Scientific Research in London. He was a member of the Pharmaceutical Society of Great Britain and also lectured at the Physicians and Surgeons College of Microbiology, London. He was a director of the Jumel Laboratories for Scientific Research in New York, where he also served as the national secretary for the Health Education Society. This society, which Empringham founded in 1926, offered inexpensive medical care in New York City. The staff of physicians and trained nurses visited homes, instructing people in health, hygiene, and disease prevention.

At a young age, a physician diagnosed Empringham as having a degenerative condition that caused him to appear much older than his chronological age. The doctor told him,

> You are an old man. Senility is not a question of the calendar — not a mere matter of the number of years since we came into the world. The degenerated condition of the body called "old age" [sic] is merely a register of the damage that has been done to our organs and tissues by various poisons. You have the worst case of intestinal toxemia I have seen in a man of your years.[7]

This prognosis was confirmed by other specialists, and Empringham was not given long to live. At the time of Empringham's prognosis, Metchnikoff had just startled the scientific world by his discovery of the protective flora of the colon. Sick as Empringham was, he went to the Pasteur Institute to learn what he could from this great man.

One year later, as a result of his education from Metchnikoff, Empringham returned to England with his health much improved. His blood pressure was lower, and the continual intestinal distress that had tortured him night and day for years was gone. His pulse, however, was still frightfully irregular, and other bodily conditions were far from normal.

In spite of his own fragile health, Empringham desired to learn more about the role of intestinal bacteria in creating either health or disease in the body. In Paris, he had become familiar with fecal examination and techniques for culturing microorganisms. Empringham arranged to receive fecal specimens of patients in London hospitals, along with the patient case histories, from laboratories. The data thus compiled proved to him, and to the bacteriologists associated with him, that Metchnikoff's theory was correct.

Dr. Empringham discovered some of the essential factors for successful implantation of lactobacteria in the human colon. He discovered that a human strain must be utilized and that the lactobacteria must be implanted rectally for lasting results.

During the time he was involved with this research, Empringham was a chemistry and microbiology student in London. He also went back to school to learn as much as possible about the science of nutrition. He was sure that his intestinal toxemia and the many maladies that followed in the wake of his autointoxication had their origin in years of incorrect eating habits.

Dr. Empringham was his own guinea pig. For years, he kept records of each meal. Each day, and sometimes every few hours, he gave himself a complete urinalysis, fecal analysis, and blood test. In this way, he gradually identified the foods that were beneficial for him and those he should avoid. He also identified the foods that were optimal for maintaining a normal colon flora and preventing problems.

Dr. Empringham wrote several books and continued this research throughout his life. His findings and insights are extremely valuable today.

The True Fountain of Youth

These two men, Professor Eli Metchnikoff and Dr. James Empringham, sought a mechanism for prolonging the human life span and improving immune function. They found their answer in the colon. They literally discovered the true fountain of youth! Metchnikoff,

Empringham, and others found that intestinal toxemia significantly contributed to degenerative disease and shortened life expectancy.

In this century, supporting research has been contributed by scientists in the United States, Europe, India, and Japan. Since 1935, reports on this topic have appeared in such medical journals as *The New England Journal of Medicine*, *The American Journal of Clinical Nutrition*, *The Journal of Infectious Disease*, *The Lancet*, and others. There is a wealth of data from the 1970s up to the current time.

While some of the data from the earlier part of this century is outdated and no longer applicable, much of this important research remains sound in principle today. It is an unfortunate trend in medicine that any research older than one year is often considered outdated. Truth does not become outmoded in a few years or in a few generations.

CHAPTER 13

Microbiology and Colon Hygiene: A Good Marriage

The meaning of the term "colon hygiene" is exactly as it sounds. "Hygiene" is from the Greek word meaning "healthful," referring to conditions and practices conducive to health. Hygiene also means "clean" or "sanitary." Just as dental hygiene means keeping your teeth and mouth clean and clear of decay-causing bacteria, colon hygiene means cleansing the colon. It is unknown when this term first came into use, but we use it here to discuss this specialized area of practice concerned with colon health.

Colon hygiene is neither the practice of medicine, nor is it concerned with diagnosis or treatment of any disease. Colon hygiene is a preventive technique of clearing the colon in order to prevent or stop the process of autointoxication by using natural, nontoxic substances.

In the United States, the era between 1900 to 1930 saw a renewed interest in colon cleansing. During this period, colon hygiene equipment and procedures were introduced. Enema techniques were found to be limited. The equipment used for enemas allowed water to penetrate only a short distance, perhaps 24 inches into the left side of the colon. Thus, cleansing was limited to only a small portion of the colon, usually the rectum and possibly a portion of the descending colon. Other techniques, such as using a thin, 52-inch hose that was to reach the cecum, were potentially dangerous and eventually abandoned.

In the 1920s to early 1930s, interest in colon hygiene coincided with the philosophical leanings of medical practice, which emphasized focal infections as the cause of many health problems. Focal infections, located in the tonsils, nasal accessory sinuses, gallbladder, appendix, and the roots of teeth, were considered to produce secondary infections, systemic changes, or toxemia.[1] The colon, considered a chief cause of focal infections, was gaining wider recognition.

All of these factors, plus others, eventually led to the development of colonic procedure and apparatus. The colonic, though similar to the enema, used a different apparatus. While the enema only cleansed the lower part of the descending colon, the colonic, when administered properly, was capable of cleansing the whole colon to the cecum.

In 1923, Phillip Norman, M.D., invented a colonic gravity flow apparatus that he used for implanting *L. acidophilus* rectally. He believed that to obtain satisfactory results in the treatment of some colon diseases, the colon should first be cleansed of all the putrefactive material.

Dr. Norman also found exercise of the colon musculature essential for bringing the atonic type back to a proper functioning state, overcoming partial obstructions caused by adhesions, and relieving many spastic conditions. He found that when the muscle tone of the colon was poor, constipation, stagnation of the feces, and proliferation of harmful microorganisms resulted.

Also in 1923, Lieutenant H.V. Hughens, United States Navy Medical Corps, improved on Dr. Norman's colonic apparatus. Both Norman and Hughens implanted acidophilus rectally after emptying the colon. No information is available about the source of the culture used by either of these researchers. In fact, the only information given about the culture was that it was in a milk medium.

H.V. Hughens wrote the following:

> There has been much written about colon pathology, its causes and treatment. To-day [*sic*] the profession is familiar with the principal causes of pathological conditions of the colon. Prolonged error in diet takes its place as one of the most frequent underlying causes. Many colonic disturbances are, no doubt, caused by focal infection the primary site of which is located in the respiratory and upper digestive tracts

and in the sinuses. It is thought by some that the colon itself often harbors the primary focus of infection from which stubborn rheumatic, digestive, and other disturbances are manifested.

It is true that for centuries the physician has thought that many of the human ailments are caused by intestinal autointoxication. Consequently from time to time the practice has been general [sic] to purge the patient regardless of the character of his illness.

Various corrective measures have been used in the treatment of constipation, chronic and acute colitis, colonic stasis, and autointoxication; *e.g.,* agar, mineral oil, combinations of mineral oil and agar, exercises of various kinds, and dietetic measures. Some have used "high enemas" of astringent and antiseptic solutions. Surgery of the colon is being practiced. All these have been disappointing.

At the present time the profession is flooded with remedies for the cleansing of the intestinal tract and cure of the conditions mentioned above. Most of these remedies are palliative and produce no permanent good results. On the other hand, cathartics cause many patients to become habitual users. The habitual use of cathartics contributes toward the production of a chronic inflammatory condition of the intestinal tract, especially the colon, with which goes, of course, a chronic infection.[2]

In 1925, Hughens went on to write:

The cases described in this article are typical of the limited number treated by the writer by the procedure given. All were markedly improved or cured. Since July, 1923, the experience of the writer in using the procedure described has been so gratifying that he takes this opportunity to recommend its use in hospitals, where complete data can be kept and close observation of the patients is practicable.[3]

Unfortunately, this sage recommendation of H.V. Hughens in 1925 was never taken up by any doctors or hospitals. It is fascinating to think what a different course the history of medicine could have taken if this procedure had been recognized for its worth. However, research into replacing the normal colon flora slowed down in early 1940, when antibiotic use became widespread, as the germ theory of disease and the philosophy of the magic bullet were almost universally adopted.

In the initial excitement of a new discovery that gave miraculous results, replacement therapy was not pursued by the scientific community as vigorously as it once was. Instead, medicine went the technological route, developing drugs and protocols for the growing onslaught of degenerative diseases and traumatic injuries, achieving a high success rate in these areas. However, the truly preventive nature of medicine left the realms of allopathic medicine and has yet to return.

Colon hygiene offers true prevention, but only when performed correctly and in accord with scientific knowledge. It is possible that microbiological knowledge during Hughens' time was insufficient for the medical community to recognize the importance of a healthy colon flora.

Hughens and Norman were the first in Western medical history to put two branches of science together (microbiology and colon hygiene). They realized the strength and implications of such a union. Only when colon hygiene is combined with microbiology can we enter the 21st century with a truly effective method of colon hygiene.

CHAPTER 14

A Giant Step Backward

B ecause modern medicine abandoned the scientific advance-
ment of colon hygiene, years of accumulated knowledge fell
by the wayside. The human concern with health and hygiene persisted, and so did the ideas of colon cleansing, enemas, and colonics.
These all then fell into the realm of the layperson, who developed
procedures that were not based on any scientific principles or knowledge. In this lay population, traces of colon hygiene have survived —
just barely. In its present state, colon hygiene is based on incomplete
and often erroneous information, the consequences of medical aban-
donment.

Colon Hygiene in the 1990s

Colon hygiene, as it exists today, is practiced with a simplistic approach and no knowledge of colon ecology or microbiology. The current methods are similar to those used in the 1800s, prior to the
microbiological findings of Metchnikoff and the practical applications
of Norman and Hughens. Colon hygienists use any one of a variety of
apparatus to introduce plain water and other substances into the colon to flush out the waste material. This is generally done in a series
of 10 or more colonics, at a rate of one to three per week.

No standard guidelines govern this procedure, and the type of
apparatus used varies widely. The use of some outdated types, such
as gravity flow equipment, should be reconsidered. The type of apparatus used and the degree of hygiene observed are not to be under-
estimated, as these factors influence the effectiveness and outcome
of the procedure.

The FDA has approved certain colon hygiene apparatus, functionally the safest and most modern in design, but some practitioners still use non-approved instruments.

Colon disease has not decreased in the world population despite efforts to drive toxins out of the colon with water colonic irrigations. Some of the chemicals and medications used in these purging procedures can be detrimental, and not only to the microorganisms. The drama escalates as people believe they need to cleanse their colon by some method for the rest of their lives. They either read books about colon hygiene, listen to someone in the field of colon hygiene, or hear from a friend-of-a-friend that they must detox, detox, detox!

The reason for continued suffering is incomplete knowledge. A little information in this field is about as good as none at all — and perhaps worse. A wise man once said, "It does not matter if a man has a thousand followers if he does not know the way!"

In most cases, water colonics, when administered correctly, do provide relief because they are effective in removing impactions. At times, water colonics have helped people overcome their suffering when nothing else would. However, water colonics have serious drawbacks that must be considered. Most importantly, water colonics are an incomplete method that leaves the colon in an alkaline state and does not address re-establishment of the natural, healthy colon flora.

Many colon hygienists add substances to their procedure that have no scientific basis. For example, some people administer "oxygen colonics," where pure oxygen is mixed with the water entering the colon. Oxygen, as an additive for colon hygiene procedures, is a completely unfounded procedure. Since the colon is naturally an anaerobic tube (lacking oxygen), why should oxygen be injected into the water during or at the end of a colonic session?

According to the proponents of this procedure, oxygen destroys bacteria and parasites that are anaerobes, those that live in the absence of oxygen. Beneficial colon bacteria, such as *L. acidophilus,* which are anaerobic, require virtually no oxygen for survival. Oxygen will kill these beneficial lactobacteria. The few sparse aerobic bacteria that do exist in the colon help foster this oxygen-free, ideal environment for the anaerobic bacteria by consuming any minute amount of oxygen that may be produced.[1] Oxygen colonics, as do antibiotics, kill both good and bad bacteria indiscriminately, leaving the colon in an alkaline condition. Any possible benefit to this procedure does not justify the risk.

Other additives are often used during the irrigation process or at the end of a session. These include coffee, wheat grass, herbs, vegetable oils, ozone, or hydrogen peroxide. None of these substances creates conditions favorable to a slightly acidic colon pH, in which the lactobacteria can establish. They all leave the colon in an alkaline condition, providing the perfect medium for the proliferation of harmful microorganisms.

Another drawback of current colonic procedures is that 10 or more sessions are required. This places excessive stress on the colon tissues, wall, and musculature. Some people claim to have had as many as 100 colonics. The only reason so many sessions are given is because the current techniques are incomplete and do not provide a means for adjusting and maintaining the colon at the correct pH. After a colonic that does not establish proper pH, the beneficial bacteria will not be able to reestablish themselves.

Even after as many as 10 or more water colonic sessions, some clients have commented that their colon was still not emptied completely. This is due to two factors. First, the colon naturally fills with waste as one eats. To achieve best results, it is necessary to clear the colon completely to the cecum. With sessions scheduled every other day or even weekly, this is not possible. Secondly, the colon must be emptied using a specific procedure, including acidifying the colon to ensure the colon's return to a healthy state.

Many individuals are dependent on colonics simply because the current procedures offered have no lasting results. For similar reasons, others overuse home enemas, or purchase home units that attach to the toilet to self-administer high enemas.

Colon Cleansers

An old practice still popular among health practitioners and laypeople alike is the use of colon cleansers or laxatives to move the bowels. The average person today uses laxatives excessively to the detriment of their health. Although these laxative products are not intended for daily or long-term use, most of them are being used in just that manner.

Many herbal colon cleansers on the market contain senna, rhubarb, cascara sagrada, or other herbs that irritate the colon lining. These herbs are meant for only occasional use in extreme conditions. All colon cleansers provide only temporary symptomatic relief. The underlying cause of poor elimination, an incorrect colon pH, is not being addressed. Continued ingestion of deficient diets, along with overuse of laxative products, only makes the problem worse.

One of the most widely used cleansers is psyllium. In the past 10 years, as people have sought to resolve their mounting colon problems, psyllium has become popular. When allowed to sit in a glass of water, psyllium turns into a thick, slimy, gelatinous substance. It absorbs 40 times its weight in water!

To consider the effect of this, remember that the colon is an absorption chamber. In the healthy system, when food residues empty through the ileocecal valve into the cecum, the residue is in a soft, liquid form. As the absorption process continues, the residue travels through the five-foot length of colon, and the feces become more dry and solid. Water and valuable electrolytes are reabsorbed back into the body. Psyllium can cause too much water absorption in the colon and can contribute to fecal impaction.

In a recent study, 24 healthy men over the age of 18 were given psyllium to test its cholesterol-lowering effect. These men had normal body weight, no disease, and were not taking any medications. The men reported the following adverse effects from ingesting psyllium: lower intestinal gas, indigestion, abdominal cramping, rectal pain, and diarrhea.[2]

I have seen many psyllium users complain of having no elimination for 7 to 10 days, fatigue, lower-back pain, constipation, and gas. They were no less than astonished to learn that what they thought was their top-notch cleanser had actually worsened their condition. Thirty percent of my scheduled appointments are made by people who have taken psyllium in some form. Psyllium, in small amounts, may be beneficial for a few people when used sparingly, but when used regularly or over the long term, it is a severe impediment to colon health.

The professional athlete who sought my services for an emergency appointment is a classic example of the psyllium syndrome. He was in his mid-30s and had begun to ingest psyllium daily (one table-spoon in eight ounces of water, increasing consumption by one table-spoon per day) to clean his colon for better athletic performance. Previously, he had regular elimination every day. During the time he began ingesting psyllium, he made no dietary changes.

By the fifth day, he was ingesting five tablespoons of psyllium and had experienced no elimination. He assumed he needed more psyllium. He was experiencing severe back pain when he came slowly walking into my office. Seventy-five minutes into the colon hygiene procedure, 10 inches of solid psyllium mass began to move out of his colon. His relief was pronounced, and he declared that he had no idea what he could have done to remove the problem on his own.

Another product used for cleansing is bentonite, which also has strong powers of absorption. Bentonite, a rock composed of clay minerals, is marketed in a powder or liquid form. Chemically, it is known as hydrated aluminum silicate.[3] Insoluble in water, it will swell to about 12 times its size when added to water.

People use bentonite because it claims to cleanse the colon and pull out all toxins, eliminating them from the body. Since bentonite has an alkaline pH, it cannot adjust the colon pH to the appropriate acid level; thus, use of bentonite cannot contribute to lasting colon health.

In the past 25 years, sensational pictures of so-called impactions in the colon have circulated throughout the health field. Some pictures depict hardened, black masses several feet long, supposedly evacuated from the colon and often still in the shape of the colon. Those circulating these pictures state that fecal matter becomes encrusted on the colon wall and forms a solid mass of black matter that must be shed, much like a snake sheds its skin.

These pictures have caused fear and uneasiness in the public. A person whose colon was near this type of condition would more likely be found in the obituary column than at a cleansing retreat.

Most of the pictures of colon impactions are from people who have allegedly gone through rigorous cleansing programs before eliminating the black encrustations. Such programs included ingesting substances such as psyllium and bentonite. My theory is that using these substances possibly contributes to the formation of encrustations if, in fact, they exist at all. When the colon is already filled with alkaline, putrefactive waste, added bulk such as psyllium and bentonite can actually make the situation worse.

If you consult gastroenterologists who use fiber optic cameras in the colon, you will be told that they rarely, if ever, see anything as extreme as portrayed in these pictures. Never have I seen or experienced anything like this in my years of experience with colon hygiene.

To date, no reliable information has been available to educate the public about colon health care. A plethora of laxative products and colon cleansers is available in both drug and health food stores, where they are top sellers. People have fallen prey to misinformation, myths, and ineffective treatments because they have been relentlessly seeking relief from constipation, diarrhea, or flatulence. The root cause of all these discomforts is an alkaline colon pH. The essential factor has been overlooked, which is replacement of the normal lactobacteria colon flora.

Another product group that is a top seller in health food stores is acidophilus supplements. Again, people are using these products under the mistaken impression this will help them achieve colon health. Misinformation about acidophilus products is so rampant, I devote a whole chapter to this subject.

CHAPTER 15

Setting the Record Straight: The Definitive Report on Lactobacteria

Almost everyone has heard of acidophilus, the friendly bacteria. Acidophilus is considered synonymous with colon health. Laypeople and health practitioners alike consider acidophilus supplementation to be the panacea for colon problems.

Many nutritionally conscious medical doctors prescribe acidophilus supplements and yogurt for their patients after a course of antibiotics, as do natural health practitioners. These health care providers are all under the mistaken impression that acidophilus is a new magic bullet for post-antibiotic care and other syndromes. In fact, this is not so.

"Acidophilus" has come to be used as a generic term for all lactobacteria. Technically, however, it refers specifically to the beneficial bacterium, *Lactobacillus acidophilus*, which is the most well-known lactobacteria species.

According to *Mosby's Medical & Nursing Dictionary*, "*Lactobacillus* means any one of a group of nonpathogenic, Gram-positive, rod-shaped bacteria that produce lactic acid from carbohydrates."[1] *Bifidobacteria* belong to the Actinomycetales subbranch of Gram-positive bacteria.

These and other bacteria that produce lactic acid are considered the beneficial bacteria.[2] They are sensitive to oxygen and moisture and, consequently, must be cultured and packaged properly to be viable for commercial use.

Lactobacteria Standards

In 1980, only five or six lactobacteria products made for oral consumption were available to the consumer. According to the retail industries *Whole Food Source Book* in 1993, 120 products were listed, not including those sold exclusively by health professionals. In fact, many of the products sold by health professionals are identical to those that can be purchased in the health food store, differing only in label and price.

Lactobacteria products are offered in every imaginable permutation: different ingredients and fillers; chewable, powder, or liquid forms; with or without lactose; vegetarian, and tempting flavors. In the past 100 years, just about every idea has been used to give health professionals, retailers, and consumers the hope that by oral ingestion, lactobacteria will implant in the colon.

In 1899, Eli Metchnikoff applied what he called "replacement therapy" when he experimented with implanting *Lactobacillus bulgaricus*, a beneficial lactobacteria, in the colon to eliminate harmful disease-forming species. Ever since this first unsuccessful experiment, replacement therapy has been a major area of interest in the quest for colon health.

Today, much more research is available on this subject. Applying this knowledge about the colon lactobacteria allows us to understand which therapies or products are useful and which are not. Certain questions must be asked and answered to see what will stand up to inquiry in the light of day and what will not.

The term "probiotic" literally means "for life," in contrast to "antibiotic," which means "against life." "Probiotic" is a recent word, coined in the mid-1970s, with the upsurge in lactobacteria products on the market. A general term, it refers to lactobacteria and other bacteria that help the host by promoting health.

In 1989, the National Nutritional Foods Association (NNFA) adopted a labeling standard for probiotics. However, this standard does not include identifying whether the source of the lactobacteria is human or animal, which is an unfortunate oversight. Only human-source lactobacteria will take up residence in and benefit the human colon. (This is discussed further in Chapter 16.) To find out if the source of your lactobacteria product is human or animal, ask your retailer or call the company yourself.

Route of Ingestion

A post-antibiotic method is absolutely necessary to re-implant and reestablish the lost beneficial colon flora. Today, no such method exists on a widely available scale. Many physicians and laypeople are under the impression that oral ingestion of lactobacteria achieves such long-term colonization. There are simply no results to substantiate this claim in the adult human colon.

Nonetheless, almost everyone is under the illusion that we need only to ingest one of the multitude of available lactobacteria-containing products. Presto! The trillions of beneficial bacteria will then overcome some two pounds (or about one-third of total fecal weight) of putrefactive alkaline bacteria in the colon, transform the pH to normal, and maintain normal pH from that moment on.

This is like sowing seeds on unfertilized, unhealthy soil. There will simply be no germination.

Orally ingested lactobacteria will not transform the colon flora. The oral route is not an effective method of implanting or reestablishing the colon lactobacteria. If it were, millions of consumers would have experienced an end to their suffering and there would have been no impetus for me to develop the technique that achieves what oral ingestion does not.

Ironically, many trillions of lactobacteria have been sold over the past 50 years, as the frequency of colon problems continues to rise. Oral ingestion of lactobacteria does not and will not re-establish the normal flora. Little, if any, orally-ingested lactobacteria actually reach the colon. The small amount that may reach the colon will be ineffective at transforming the flora.

In order for oral ingestion to be effective, the bacteria must survive first the stomach's strong acids and then the small intestine's alkaline environment. Lactobacteria are not equipped to survive either of these pH conditions. The stomach's pH range, as we saw in Chapter 2, is from 1.5 (very acidic) to 3.0 (medium acidic), depending on the stage of digestion. Beyond the duodenum, the normal pH of the small intestine is 6.5 to 7.5. How will the lactobacteria survive the transit through these two hostile territories?

Depending on the source you consult, you will see recommendations that children and adults ingest lactobacteria either before, with, between, or after meals. The proposed rationale for this advice is that the stomach's hydrochloric acid has been sufficiently diluted with food to change the very acidic pH to a less acidic pH. In theory, this less acidic pH will not antagonize the lactobacteria, and they will travel safely to the colon.

Consider that lactobacteria thrive only in a slightly acidic environment, in the pH range of 6.4 to 4.5. Growth of the lactobacteria ceases when the acidic pH of 4.0 to 3.6 is reached, depending on the species and strain.[3] How then will they survive the stomach's digestive pH, which is over 10 times more acidic than the pH at which they cease to grow?

In 1891, Sir Frederick Grant Banting, a Canadian physiologist, professor, and one of the principle discoverers of insulin, realized the strength of stomach acid when he found the path that insulin travels from the pancreas to the bloodstream. In order to be effective, insulin had to be injected directly into the muscle, bypassing the strong stomach acid.

Likewise, when viable lactobacteria (or other beneficial bacteria) are taken orally as a food or a supplement, they will not survive the strong acid of the healthy adult stomach. Note that the stomach of breastfed infants is not highly acidic. Stomach conditions are quite different in the infant than in the adult.

Human lactobacteria must be implanted directly in the human colon and will only stay alive when the colon has been initially emptied of any toxic contents, and the proper slightly-acid pH has been established.

The following study is from promotional material distributed to consumers by Kovac Laboratories, Inc., around 1980. Kovac Laboratories had been in business more than 40 years and pioneered the first human-source liquid *L. acidophilus* sold in health food stores.

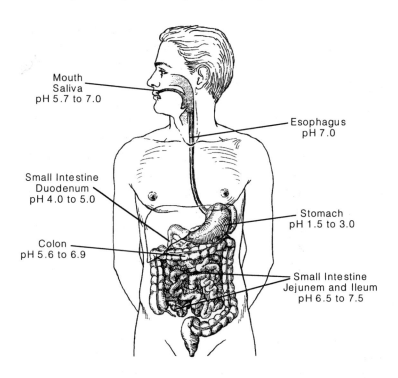

Mouth
Saliva
pH 5.7 to 7.0

Esophagus
pH 7.0

Small Intestine
Duodenum
pH 4.0 to 5.0

Stomach
pH 1.5 to 3.0

Colon
pH 5.6 to 6.9

Small Intestine
Jejunem and Ileum
pH 6.5 to 7.5

Lactobacteria optimum range: pH 6.4 to 4.5

Lactobacteria growth ceases at: pH 4.0 to 3.6

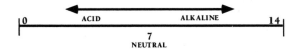

Figure 8. Lactobacteria pH Relative to Digestive pH[4,5]

An independent laboratory tested several brands of *L. acidophilus* drinks in a simulated stomach fluid with a pH of 1.2, the theoretical acidity at which humans digest protein. The initial shock of exposure to pH 1.2 killed from 40% to 70% of the bacteria immediately. The loss after an additional 30 minutes was another 10%.[6]

Morning Star Laboratories, Inc., in Simi Valley, California, did the following experiment.[7] They placed two strains, *L. acidophilus* and *B. bifidum,* in separate solutions of normal stomach acid for 30 minutes. None survived the stomach's hydrochloric acid, which normally sterilizes bacteria on food we ingest to protect us from infection by many types of microbes.

Some manufacturers of lactobacteria products explain that since their products are enteric coated (a protective coating to allow pills or capsules to pass through the digestive tract), they can successfully implant in the colon. In order to implant, the enteric products must pass through the stomach acid, bile, trypsin, and 14 feet of digested foodstuff in the small intestine.

If a few lactobacteria do manage to escape devastation by stomach acid, they are confronted with bile in the upper small intestine. Bile has an antibacterial effect and is responsible for the low transit numbers of bacteria in the healthy small intestine.[8] Due to bile and other digestive secretions in the small intestine, the pH remains quite alkaline, which again is detrimental to our lactobacteria friends.

Let us presume the best scenario for this transit. Most lactobacteria are indeed killed, but a few survive the worst pH extremes. Like determined travelers, these lactobacteria survive the coldest winter and cross the hottest desert. When they finally reach their homeland, they find it overrun by trillions of hostile invaders. How can they take back their country? There are not enough of them.

Similarly, the arrival of a few billion lactobacteria in an alkaline colon is not sufficient to overcome the pathogens and transform the alkaline colon to a slightly acidic pH. The acid-loving lactobacteria will not survive, let alone implant, in an alkaline environment. They will be outnumbered and overwhelmed by the resident pathogens and yeasts of the alkaline colon. It is like sending a few Boy Scouts to fight a major war where the enemy already commands the territory.

Space in the colon is limited, and the predominant, pathology-causing microorganisms are not going to give up their established territory.[9] In order for lactobacteria to be able to tip the scales under these conditions, the scales must already be largely in their favor. As evidenced by the fact that *Taber's Medical Dictionary* considers an

Whenever you hear about a certain product or therapy, ask the following questions:

- What effect will it have on the colon pH?

- What will it do to reacidify the colon?

- What effects will it have on the lactobacteria colon flora?

- Will it survive the stomach acids, bile, and trypsin to reach the colon?

- Does it achieve lasting results in the colon?

- What data is there to substantiate the claims?

- Is the data based on human, in vivo, studies?

- What is the source of the lactobacteria?

Table 3. Assessing Colon Treatments and Products

alkaline colon "normal," the chances of this are very slim. Thus, the whole concept of oral implantation makes no rational sense whatsoever.

In a 1984 study, two strains of human *L. acidophilus* in milk were administered to individuals with no evidence that the intestine was permanently colonized with these strains.[10] A similar result was seen in a study that showed implantation of human *L. acidophilus* does not occur in the gastrointestinal tract of healthy men who orally ingest high doses.[11]

Transformation of the alkaline human colon can only be achieved through correcting the problem at its source, through the most direct route, the rectum.

Lactobacteria for the Small Intestine?

Some lactobacteria products are said to target the small intestine.

However, efforts to colonize the small intestine with lactobacteria are futile. Remember, most of the small intestine has an alkaline pH for assimilating nutrients and contains some oxygen; the few aerobic types of bacteria existing in the small intestine are transients. The small intestine is not a favorable medium for the anaerobic, acid-loving lactobacteria that primarily exist in the absence of oxygen.

The small intestine is subdivided into three parts: the duodenum, the jejunum, and the ileum. In health, the first 8 to 11 inches of the small intestine, the duodenum, is almost completely sterile.[12] The pH of the duodenum is acid, ranging between pH 4 and 5. The distance from the duodenum to the ileum is about 14 feet. In this length, an increase to alkaline pH takes place. The sparse microbial inhabitants of the region are transient only and may or may not be alive. Here the cell count of bacteria is small, with the population ranging between 100 thousand to 10 million per gram of digestive material in the lower ileum.[13]

The healthy small intestine is sterile, which means free of living organisms.[14] Studies show the small intestine to contain very few bacteria. These transients pass through with the digesting food and are not resident bacteria colonizing the tract. Finally, microorganisms must successfully overcome many obstacles to colonize epithelial surfaces in the healthy small intestine.[15]

It becomes clear that anaerobic lactobacteria are normally meant to colonize only the lower part of the gastrointestinal tract, the colon, and not the small intestine. The small intestine functions as a true organ of digestion and assimilation. The colon, however, is meant to function as an anaerobic fermentative chamber, filled with lactobacteria flora that maintain a slightly acidic pH. This condition creates maximum health.

All efforts to restore the colon to health using laxatives, colon cleansers, or oral lactobacteria supplements are futile. Two essential factors have been overlooked: reacidification of the colon and reestablishment of the normal lactobacteria colon flora.

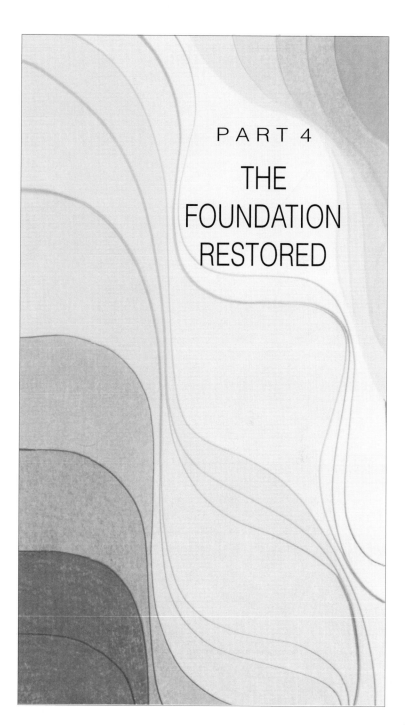

PART 4

THE
FOUNDATION
RESTORED

CHAPTER 16

Webster Implant Technique: Colon Hygiene into the 21st Century

L et us say that we are in charge of tending a healthy organic garden. In ignorance, we inadvertently change the normal, slightly acid pH of the soil to an alkaline pH. This change causes a chain reaction. First, soil nutrients will no longer be assimilated well, causing the plants to degenerate. Next, weeds, parasites, and fungi will soon destroy the garden and no room will remain for flowers or crops to grow.

The colon is the soil of the body. At this juncture in history, the colon flora has been devastated, leaving our immunity at a low ebb and our systems open to invasion and overgrowth of harmful micro-organisms. When the lactobacteria, our protective shield, have been suppressed or inadvertently destroyed, they must be reestablished. While many have realized this necessity, all attempts to date have proven ineffective.

Scientists, microbiologists, researchers, and laypeople around the world have all found different pieces of the puzzle. Over the past 100 years, it has been the microbiologists who have realized the importance and uniqueness of the colon flora. Physicians acknowledge the necessity of replacing the flora after antibiotic therapy. Colon therapists know that colon hygiene is an important part of health. But, until now, these diverse areas of research, expertise, and clinical practice have not been united.

All attempts at oral implantation have proven unsuccessful and incomplete. Perhaps now we are ready to take a new approach. The only route for effective reimplantation of the healthy colon flora is the rectal route, using human-source lactobacteria.

Webster Implant Technique (WIT), evolved from the research explored in this book, offers a complete procedure to restore a healthy colon environment. Over the past two decades of my research and experience, colon hygiene has been reinvented and aligned with modern microbiological and scientific knowledge. This synthesis of old wisdom and new information provides a complete approach to colon hygiene that is gentle, safe, and effective.

WIT has been provided to over 1,500 clients in six years of clinical practice. It reestablishes the lactobacteria colon flora and slightly acidic colon pH, which are the foundation of health in the body. We have seen that water colonics clear impactions, but do not stop toxic production. Water colonics do not address the cause, which is why the procedure has never really caught on.

All attempts at colon cleansing without restoring the slightly acidic pH of the colon are incomplete. It is like deciding to remodel your house. After you have taken everything apart and have cleaned every room in your house, are you done? Certainly not! The goal of remodeling is to make your house better than it was before, not just throw everything away or patch it up. You want to move back in to a better house, right? Design in hand, you have it remodeled. You make sure the foundation and structure are sound, you paint, and soon you can move your things back in and be better for it. Then you have to keep the place up.

It is the same in the colon. Just cleansing the colon is like clearing everything out of your house and leaving your house empty. You can't live like that. You need to replenish your colon flora, which is like giving your house a good foundation and moving all the useful items back in their place. Now you have a pleasant and functional home, or a healthy and thriving colon flora.

Webster Implant Technique

For 90% of people, WIT can be completed in two one-hour sessions, two days in a row. The other 10% may require three sessions. The total colon will empty in two or three sessions. Less than 5% of people need to return for repeat treatments, showing the efficiency of this unique technique.

WIT is very effective in loosening solid waste because whey in the water begins to acidify the colon right away. Production of toxins in the colon ceases as the colon pH is normalized. This relieves the whole system and allows toxins a way out via the portal vein, liver, blood, kidneys, bladder, and skin. As the system detoxifies, balance can become a reality. The goal is to achieve a healthy colon in the most efficient manner and then to get on with life.

There is a pandemic colon problem on this planet at present. When this complete procedure is performed correctly, more people can be helped.

WIT Procedure

WIT has become more widely accepted, and many practitioners have begun to offer "acidophilus implants" because of client requests. However, WIT cannot be successfully practiced by someone without specialized training. When implantation is done with incomplete knowledge, effectiveness is diminished.

I have had laypeople experience my procedure once or twice and then open their own business, representing WIT as their work or claiming to have trained with me. People have come to me after seeing these technicians and experiencing no lasting results. In the long run, no one benefits by this type of ineffective practice.

Simply reading this book will not qualify someone to practice this technique correctly, as many aspects cannot be mentioned here. Training is essential so the practitioner understands the proper condition of a healthy colon. When different situations arise in practice, appropriate action can be taken based on a firm foundation of knowledge.

Ideally, colon hygiene should be administered by a licensed health professional with a working understanding of anatomy, microbiology, and basic science. A practitioner who is experimenting and performing a purely mechanical technique is not qualified. The colon hygienist must be an educated and highly informed participant, not merely a technician.

At present, no individual other than myself has been trained to administer WIT. Registered nurses, as a group, are perhaps the best qualified to learn this procedure, as they have adequate training to grasp the microbiological implications that are a critical aspect of this work.

WIT should not be performed in hospitals due to the presence of *Staphylococcus*, *Streptococcus*, and other microorganisms, which would interfere with achieving clear, consistent results through contamination and infection. WIT should be performed in a clinical setting in an office used only for this purpose.

Water pressure is an important aspect of colon cleansing. A very low, gentle, controlled pressure is not only the safest, it achieves the best results. Excessive water pressure is absolutely unnecessary when a colonic is administered properly. With low pressure and correct manipulation of modern equipment, the waste will be gently evacuated with maximum comfort and relaxation for the client. Only colon hygiene equipment that is registered with the Food and Drug Administration should be used.

Only purified water can be used for the procedure. It must be free of chlorine, lead, asbestos, pesticides, other contaminants, and microorganisms. Recently, several cities have reported contamination of their water supply with small parasites such as *Cryptosporidium,* while other areas may contain *Giardia* in their water supply. Precaution is the best measure.

Four Steps to a Healthy Colon

Most methods to date have tried to implant the colon using a one-step method, but there are many essential factors that must coexist simultaneously to reestablish and then support the lactobacteria colon flora. There are four steps required to successfully reestablish the healthy colon flora.

First, the colon is cleansed of accumulated waste and toxins all the way to the cecum. This is like clearing your yard of noxious weeds so you can plant a garden. Second, the colon is gently re-acidified, which is like preparing the soil to plant a garden. Third, a viable strain of high-quality human lactobacteria is implanted rectally into the colon. This is like planting flower seeds in your garden. Fourth, the colon flora is nourished and maintained, just as you would water and give nutrients to your garden plants.

Step One: Cleanse

The long-held tenet that the colon is both the root of disease in the body and also the potential fountain of youth is confirmed by research over the last 100 years. Evidence links toxins manufactured in the colon to serious disease conditions in the body. The main route of transmission, as we have seen, is from the colon, through the mesenteric veins, to the portal vein, and hence to the liver. When the liver is either overwhelmed by toxins or unable to process them, the toxins enter the bloodstream and begin to affect other organs and tissues of the body. Which areas are affected depends on many factors. Usually the weakest areas will become affected first.

A plot of land filled with noxious weeds or stripped of topsoil and nutrients due to abuse and neglect must first be cleared and tilled. It is the same with the colon. Cleansing the colon properly is essential to prepare for the lactobacteria implant. It also helps to relieve the excess toxic burden on the liver.

Step Two: Reacidify

Now that the colon, our garden plot, is cleared, the soil can be prepared. Since lactobacteria will not take hold or thrive in anything but a slightly acidic pH, something must be done to acidify the colon before the lactobacteria can successfully be implanted. This is accomplished by using a specially prepared whey wash that reacidifies the colon while assisting the breakup and elimination of impacted, putrefactive fecal matter.

Step Three: Implant

Once the colon has been emptied and slightly reacidified, a bacterial culture is rectally implanted. Great care is required to ensure that specific criteria are met in selecting a strain of bacteria. If any one of these criteria is lacking, the implant will not be successful.

Lactobacteria products may come in powder, liquid, or tablet form and contain different ingredients or fillers. Some products include lactose, others do not. Tempting flavors are added to many products. All of these factors influence the product's ability to rectally implant in the human colon.

Most products focus on claims of viability, bacteria count, and how their product reaches the colon. While these are all necessary concerns, the source of the lactobacteria is even more important, as it is a major factor in achieving lasting results.

The original experiments of Eli Metchnikoff with *Lactobacillus* failed largely because the strain he used was of bovine origin, which will not implant in the human colon.[1] Many authorities have established that only human-source lactobacteria will stay alive in the human colon.[2] Each species has its own unique strain of lactobacteria. This species specificity is a biological mechanism that protects the unique pH and biochemistry of plants, birds, and animals.[3]

Since bovine (cow) sources of bacteria are hardy, they are easier and more cost-effective to produce. For this reason, most companies use these strains in their lactobacteria products. According to Dr. Empringham, commercial firms use bovine *L. bulgaricus* because it grows rapidly in milk, thus allowing high culture counts to be claimed. However, these bovine-derived strains will not implant and take up residence in the human colon even if they are rectally implanted in a clean, empty, and slightly acid colon.

Studies show bacterial adherence to be cell-specific. *Lactobacilli* from a species will adhere best to epithelial cells from the same species and is even anatomically site-specific.[4]

Several years ago, the chief executive officer of a large company asked me to comment on their new lactobacteria product, which was still in the production phase. The first question I asked him was, "What is the source of lactobacteria? Human, plant, or bovine?"

He answered, "What difference does it make?"

It makes every difference in the world!

	Healthy Stool	Unhealthy Stool
pH	slightly acidic	alkaline
Predominant Populations	lactobacteria	pathogens
Odor	none	foul or strong odor
Color	medium brown	chalky, black, dark brown, gray
Form	well formed	loose, stringy, hard balls
Buoyancy	floats most of the time	seldom or never floats
Pattern	consistent	inconsistent
Regularity	1 to 2 times a day	less than once a day or more than 3 times a day
Other factors	no mucous, blood, or undigested food particles	presence of blood, mucous, or undigested food particles

Table 4. A Healthy and Unhealthy Stool

Step Four: Maintenance

When new grass seeds are planted, it may take 10 days before a slight, green, sprouting ground cover can be seen. In the next 20 days or so, the lawn is up and ready to walk on without being damaged. Similarly, lactobacteria, once implanted in the human colon, need time to colonize the colon.

Microorganisms encounter certain obstacles in their effort to successfully colonize epithelial surfaces. Unidirectional flow of fluids over epithelial surfaces may sweep away bacteria not firmly attached. This flow of fluids includes that caused by normal peristaltic action.

Other obstacles to colonization include epithelial cell turnover, localized immune responses, the presence of microbial competitors or antimicrobial agents and variations of pH.[5]

During each session, clients are educated about how to maintain their colon health after leaving the office so they will have no need for further colonics. Everyone is discouraged from further use of laxatives or enemas. Clients are taught practical information they can apply in their daily life to monitor and maintain their healthy colon flora.

People can easily be educated on how to observe their stools to roughly determine the pH range of their stool. Generally, a medium-brown, well-formed, floating stool with no odor signifies the presence of a healthy, slightly acidic colon pH and the predominance of a lactobacteria-type flora. (In rare cases, a floating stool can signify a fat metabolism disorder known as steatorrhea.) A sinking, dark-colored stool with a bad or foul odor guarantees the existence of an alkaline colon.

Many people are unaware that their stool should have no bad odor. A malodorous stool is perhaps the most significant factor indicating a putrefactive colon flora. Because the stool will naturally vary from day to day in accord with diet and other factors, one will not always have a perfect stool. A consistent pattern, indicating a healthy stool with slight variations but no dramatic changes, is what to look for.

The client who has received the implant must observe certain simple dietary considerations for at least one month after the procedure to ensure the growth of the implant. They can follow their normal, healthy diet, but should mainly eat foods that digest easily for them. Alcohol and red meat must be avoided for two to four weeks after receiving the implant because they can destroy the lactobacteria implant. Eggs may be eaten. Once the lactobacteria have become the dominant colon flora, small quantities of red meat or other flesh foods in the diet will not be detrimental.

Certain foods promote the growth and maintenance of lactobacteria when included in the daily diet. The relationship between food and a healthy colon flora is covered extensively in the following four chapters. Sweet dairy whey is the single most important food to promote the growth of the lactobacteria.

Who Will Benefit from WIT?

This method is a natural preventive method, not a cure. WIT will reestablish the colon flora after it is destroyed by medical or non-

No matter how many lactobacteria are introduced into the colon, if the conditions are not favorable, they will rapidly die. The following conditions are favorable to their growth:

- Anaerobiosis
- A pH value between 5.0 and 7.0
- A fermentable sugar or other source of energy
- An assimilable source of nitrogen (*e.g.*, a protein hydrolysate)
- Necessary growth factors
- Necessary minerals and trace elements

Other factors in the colon that may affect growth are:

- Surface tension
- Presence of antibiotics or other substances.

Notes:

- Given the conditions listed above, lactobacteria can ferment sugars (most notably lactose) to produce acid and create the environment favorable for themselves in the colon.

- The only common sugars that can pass through the stomach into the colon in any quantity are lactose and dextrin.

Table 5. Conditions Favorable for Proliferation of Lactobacteria in the Colon[6]

medical conditions. WIT is invaluable as a post-antibiotic therapy for either replacing the normal flora or as a procedure in cases where the colon flora is abnormal. Reestablishing the normal, beneficial bacteria addresses a major cause of disease instead of treating the symptoms.

In today's age of industrialization, there are very few people who do not have an abnormal alkaline pH in their colon. Substances that will devastate the colon flora include use and overuse of antibiotics, many pharmaceutical and nonprescription drugs, hard street drugs, birth control pills, steroids, laxatives, alcohol, excess fat or protein consumption, high stress, trauma, and injury.

By normalizing the colon pH and flora, WIT helps prevent relapse from conditions such as candidiasis and other parasitic infections, but only after these organisms have been eliminated. First, the majority of *Candida* or parasites must be destroyed. In the process of eliminating the debris that accumulates as *Candida* die off, the colon often becomes overloaded with toxic material. If the colon is not cleared and the slightly acidic pH established soon after, it will be fertile ground for another infestation. Acidifying the colon helps eliminate the debris. Establishing the lactobacteria prevents recurrence.

In order to be successful, treatment depends on the observation of rules for its correct use. Unless procedures are accurately followed, no reasonable estimate of the value of the therapy can be made, and no fair measure of success expected.

We all desire lasting results. Many individuals choose alternative therapies only after trying many different modalities. They are not interested in symptomatic relief but are looking to resolve the root cause. WIT addresses the root cause, toxic pollution in the colon, while at the same time giving the client understanding and practical information.

If colon hygiene is to survive into the 21st century and beyond, it must be updated and standardized. This means colon hygiene as it is being practiced today must completely change its approach. Common sense shows clearly that the procedure needs to be performed in accordance with modern scientific and microbiological knowledge.

Now the history of colon hygiene has been told, and the microbiological, medical, and historical endeavors are complete; the path is clear. The work that Metchnikoff began was carried on by Empringham, Norman, Hughens, and others, including myself. WIT procedure must be standardized and performed by trained clinicians who understand the implications of what they are doing. Ultimately, it may be the public who will demand this.

After all the myths and misinformation have been cleared, it is simple to see the facts that remain. As we stand at the turn of a new century, once again the principles of microbiology have been reunited with those of colon hygiene. A simple and effective procedure to restore colon health is now available. Colon hygiene practiced in such a rational manner provides a valuable tool for medicine and healing, today and in the future.

CHAPTER 17

Whey of Life

Once human strains of lactobacteria have been rectally implanted into the colon using the Webster Implant Technique (WIT), we must provide them with the sustenance for their survival. Providing implantation without providing the nutrient environment for the lactobacteria to thrive is leaving the job undone. But what is the ideal nutrient environment?

Many people have asked, "What foods should I eat to promote the growth of acidophilus?" This is a very important question.

After receiving WIT, diet influences the success of the implant. When we understand what foods benefit the lactobacteria flora, we can learn how to maintain good colon health.

Like any living organism, *Lactobacillus acidophilus* has specific dietary requirements for sustaining its life. Certain foods promote its growth, while certain foods are detrimental to its growth. Diet plays a major role in determining the type of flora that predominate in the human colon.

The two most important foods for the colon flora are whey and whole grains. These will be discussed at length. Other foods that influence colon health, for better or worse, will also be discussed.

Diet and Colon Health

Some researchers find a direct correlation between the food people eat, their colon health, and even the prevailing flora in their colon. Scientists investigating *Lactobacillus acidophilus* study its dietary and environmental requirements, metabolic patterns, and life cycle.

It is fascinating that the nutritional requirements of *Lactobacillus acidophilus* are very similar to that of humans. Like people, the primary dietary need of *L. acidophilus* is for carbohydrates. It also requires some amino acids (protein), vitamins, minerals, and a small amount of fatty acids. Human types of lactobacteria in the colon are fastidious, requiring riboflavin, niacin, pantothenate, and pyridoxine.[1]

Sweet dairy whey meets all these nutritional requirements of lactobacteria. Specifically, the most important carbohydrate required by *L. acidophilus* is lactose (milk sugar), which is most abundant in whey. Scientific studies show that if there are any lactobacteria alive in the colon, their growth can be promoted simply by providing them food. An initial dose of 240 to 400 grams of lactose was found to be effective in promoting colonization of the colon without any supplemental lactobacteria, orally or rectally.[2] Many people who do not receive WIT see beneficial results simply by including whey in their daily diet.

Another use of whey is to replenish electrolytes lost during severe dehydration. This application of whey could constitute an effective and natural means for treating diarrhea in people of all ages.[3] Diarrhea is generally due to a bacterial imbalance in the colon. When WIT is used to reestablish homeostasis (balance), whey is consumed to support the nutritional requirements of the flora, and diarrhea stops permanently. As the normal flora predominates, the colon environment can no longer support diarrhea-causing pathogens.

Whey, Sweet Whey

Just what is whey?

We are all familiar with the story of Little Miss Muffet, eating her curds and whey. In spite of our familiarity with this nursery rhyme, most of us do not know what whey is, let alone recognize it as a major contributor to human health.

Whey, the watery part of milk that is separated from the curd in the process of making cheese, is the essence of milk. All the casein and fat go into the cheese, leaving whey with no casein and a fat content equal to 1% or less. This absence of casein allows many indi-

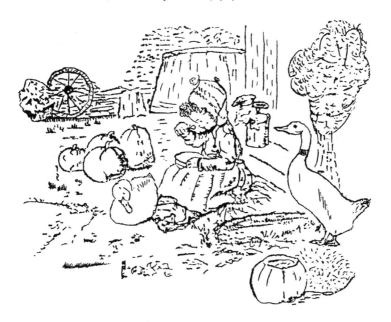

Figure 9. Little Miss Muffet sat on her tuffet,
eating her curds and whey

viduals to tolerate whey more easily than milk, since some people are allergic to casein or have trouble with the high fat content of most cheeses. Because it has no casein and virtually no fat content, whey is also very easy to digest, even for those unable to use dairy products. Whey is especially high in lactose (milk sugar).

The typical analysis of sweet whey shows it to be very good nutritionally. High in natural amino acids and minerals, it also contains some vitamins. The soluble protein lactoglobulins in whey are identical to serum globulin in human blood and contain antibodies that help strengthen the immune system.[4] The major soluble proteins in whey are beta-lactoglobulin, immunoglobulin, alpha-lactalbumin, and serum albumin.

The amino acids in whey are rated higher in bioavailability than those in eggs, according to the World Health Organization.[5] Research shows whey protein is superior to soy, rice, wheat, and beef as far as quality and bioavailability.

The pH of whey is approximately 6, which is slightly acid, ideal for gastrointestinal tract maintenance. Whey acts as a natural antiseptic, destroying or inhibiting the growth of pathogenic microorganisms while causing no harm to human tissues.

Although not included in the modern diet, whey historically made quite a contribution to the nutritional well-being of many societies. In Sweden, whey used to be included in the diet as whey cheese, whey butter, and as a whey beverage. It is no coincidence that Swedish women are world-renowned for their smooth, bright, healthy complexions.

Two centuries ago, in Scandinavia and other places in Europe, such as England, people frequented whey houses. Here, whey was freshly prepared and one could relax and enjoy rejuvenating whey drinks while socializing.

In 1850, a distinguished English physician, Thomas Sydenham, recognized the therapeutic value of whey. Dr. Sydenham is considered the founder of modern epidemiology.[6] He suggested using whey enemas and beverages to cleanse the intestinal tract of impurities.[7]

I first learned about the benefits of whey as a 10-year-old boy in California. Living within view of the Sacramento State Fairgrounds, I went to see the animals one day. I came upon some Black Angus bulls with exceptionally shiny coats and blue-ribbon awards around their necks. The farmer who had brought these prize-winning bulls to the fair was leaning against a white, wooden fence.

I asked him, "Why are your bulls so healthy with such shiny coats?"

"WHEY!" he answered. "Do you know what whey is?"

I said, "Yes. My grandmother makes cottage cheese, and it's the water she pours down the sink."

Many years later, this memory of the farmer was rekindled when I saw whey mentioned in health magazines. I began to pursue information about whey in the data banks but found only a few animal studies. When I discovered that most whey had a sour or salty and bitter taste, I realized why my grandmother poured it down the drain.

In America, whey has traditionally been used as animal feed for its nutritional value and health benefits. I later learned that some bakers use sweet whey to give pies higher quality nutrition. I spent many

Protein	Chemical Score	Biological Value*	Net Protein Value
Whey	> 100	104	92
Egg	100	94	94
Fish	71	76	80
Beef	69	74	67
Casein	58	80	72
Oats	57	65	66
Rice	56	64	57
Soybeans	47	73	61
Wheat	43	65	40
Lentils	31	45	30

*Biological Value shows the actual protein use in adults

Table 6. Comparison of Whey Protein Quality
and Bioavailability [8,9,10]

years seeking a delicious form of sweet whey made especially for human consumption.

All Whey Is Not Created Equal

There are several products that are whey protein isolates. The amino acid component of whey has been extracted, isolated, and made into a product. While these isolates may be very good as protein supplements, they are not a whole food and do not supply all the nutrients required by lactobacteria. Specifically, these protein isolates may not contain lactose, which is the primary food required by the colon lactobacteria flora.

Conversely, products that are only lactose isolates do not contain the other nutrients essential for the healthy colon lactobacteria flora. Colon function thrives when provided with whole, human-grade whey as it is made by nature because natural, whole, sweet whey is the ideal food to promote the growth of the healthy colon flora.

Whey used as a supplement for animal feed is not the same as whey processed for human use. Whey intended for human consumption is instant, sterile, and will specify that it is "Edible Grade Whey." This is a grading system used by the United States Department of Agriculture (USDA), which determines what grade will be listed on the label. The label will also state that it has been pasteurized and packaged in a state-licensed facility for good hygiene.

A Whey of Life

Over the past years, I have suggested to parents that they add sweet whey to the diet of children between 3 and 18 years of age. Within two to three weeks of incorporating one to two tablespoons daily of human-grade, good-tasting, high-quality sweet whey into their daily diet, the majority began to multiply their beneficial colon flora.

Because many children have been breastfed, their starter implant of beneficial bacteria requires only proper food to start multiplying. This is like giving the flora a "jump start" and can potentially save future generations much unnecessary suffering. Realization through education and experience will carry over to their children and create a better planet for everyone.

Adults can also follow this suggested use, but it may initially take three tablespoons daily and as long as 30 days for the beneficial bacteria, if there are any, to start multiplying and colonizing the colon. This increased consumption of whey over a longer period of time is required because of the increased height, weight, and age of adults and their state of colon health. Once regularity is realized, whey should be used as part of regular food consumption.

> **Day 1:** Mix one tablespoon of sweet whey in six ounces of water and drink on an empty stomach. This will test for any intolerance to whey. If there are no problems, such as excessive gas or discomfort, continue with directions for Day 2.

> **Day 2:** Mix two tablespoons of sweet whey in six ounces of water and drink on an empty stomach.

> **Day 3 and on:** Increase to three to four tablespoons daily until the stool becomes soft. Depending on your state of colon health, this could take 15 to 30 days.

When elimination becomes ideal, use the desired amount of whey either daily or every other day for maintenance. If the stool is too soft, use less whey. If the stool becomes too hard, increase whey. In this fashion, elimination can be regulated. When the ideal colon flora is achieved by orally consuming whey and stimulating the growth of potential latent lactobacteria, a renewed state of health will be realized.

Whey may be consumed as a delicious drink, used as a topping on fruit dishes, or added to protein drinks or yogurt shakes. As with all milk products, however, it should not be mixed with orange or other acidic fruit juices. This is not proper food combining and can contribute to digestive problems. Whey can also be added to baked goods, hot cakes, and cereal. It can be used in recipes whenever powdered milk is called for. A slight measuring adjustment may be necessary.

A True Whey Story

A mother called me after her neighbor told her of the good results she was experiencing from using sweet whey. The two ladies had been discussing colon problems in front of her nine-year-old son, who interrupted and said, "Maybe that's what I need, Mom!"

The mother called me and said her son was not able to control his colon and was having four to five spontaneous eliminations every day. She said she was at her wit's end over this problem; her son was obviously physically and emotionally uncomfortable. Over the past two years, he had been to four or five specialists in order to resolve his problem but had experienced no improvement whatsoever. She asked my advice.

I first asked her to read my booklet, *Acidophilus & Colon Health*. I then asked that she have her son stop consuming all junk food and fried food and to replace bread with Ak-Mak® whole wheat crackers. I suggested she allow her son to eat only cooked vegetables with no raw vegetables other than salad. I advised them to use cooked eggs for protein and a powdered, high-protein dairy supplement until his stool became normal. I further recommended that her son abstain from consuming meat until the colon was normal. The only fiber he was to consume was hot cereal, prepared as described in the next chapter, with sweet whey added. Until his colon normalized, he was to use whey at a concentration of one to three tablespoons per day.

Within three days, the mother called me to report that her son had stopped having so many eliminations and was feeling great. She added that she and her husband had begun to follow the same routine, and the whole family was doing better.

This is just one example of the results that can be achieved by feeding sweet whey to the lactobacteria already in the colon.

Lactose Intolerance

If you experience excessive gas during the first few days of ingesting whey, it is usually because the colon pH is reducing as its environment becomes normalized. In most cases, this is a temporary reaction and should subside in just a few days, when the normal slightly acidic pH is achieved.

If the gas does not subside or is very uncomfortable, you may be lactose intolerant. Certain people and even certain races have been shown to be genetically deficient in the enzyme *lactase*, that digests milk sugar. The suffix "-ase" is used to denote a substance that acts as an enzyme. Hence, the enzyme that works on milk sugar (lactose) is called "lactase." Some of these people, however, are able to assimilate yogurt. They will be able to utilize whey as well. In general, if you can eat yogurt, you will be able to eat whey with no problems.

Another type of lactase deficiency is found to be more puzzling. In this case, the individual does not have a genetic deficit. Very often, when this person recovers his or her normal colon flora, the enzyme lactase is again present in sufficient quantities to digest milk products.

If you suspect that you are lactose intolerant, the hydrogen breath test is a simple, noninvasive procedure used to evaluate carbohydrate absorption. This analysis specifically identifies lactose intolerance. In some people, the casein protein in dairy products is the cause of problems, not lactose. Whey is casein-free. Ask a health care professional about this simple test to eliminate guessing.

These days, it is common to hear people claim to be lactose intolerant. Many people can tolerate a small amount of whey, yogurt, or fermented milk but cannot tolerate milk. Some can use sour cream, butter, or cottage cheese, but not cheese. Supermarket shelves are now filled with dairy products that have added lactase enzyme for the purpose of helping the lactose-intolerant population break down milk sugar. The enzyme lactase is now offered in pill form. Health food stores offer an array of products that claim to be lactose-free.

Why are so many individuals unable to use milk products? Why is this such a common problem today when so many societies have been using milk products for centuries? Could antibiotics be the cause of lactase deficiency because of indiscriminate destruction of the lactose-fermenting beneficial bacteria in the colon? Could the solution for lactose intolerance be restoring the lactose-fermenting colon flora able to metabolize the malabsorbed lactose?

Bifidobacterium bifidum, the microbial species predominant in mother's breast milk, produces lactase enzymes. Most healthy, breastfed infants can digest mother's milk.

Colostrum and human milk both contain a so-called "Bifidus factor" that provides N-acetyl-D-glucosamine (NAG), promoting the growth of *B. bifidum*. *B. bifidum* is a source of the lactase enzymes required for digesting milk sugar.

According to some research, infants have trouble digesting cow's milk because this milk is low in lactase enzymes.[11] In addition, antibiotics, which have been overused in modern society, can destroy *B. bifidum*, the producers of lactase enzymes.

One excellent report points out that diarrhea in lactose-intolerant people is caused by a lactase enzyme deficiency and that lactose intolerance often decreases after long-term feeding of lactose.[12] An example of this is seen in Hawaii, where the first-generation Japanese cannot tolerate milk. As each subsequent generation is introduced to milk, their ability to digest lactose increases. This represents the multiplication of lactobacteria, producing lactase for metabolizing lactose in the colon. The amount of lactase produced is dependent on the numbers of lactobacteria.

Lactose Should Reach the Colon

There is a conceptual flaw in the practice of offering milk with added lactase enzymes to aid in the digestion of lactose for lactose-intolerant individuals. Some nutritionists believe that, due to an insufficiency of lactase, high quantities of lactose reach the colon. They believe that too much lactose in the colon is causing the digestive problems. This is not the complete picture. When insufficient quantities of lactose reach the colon, the growth of beneficial bacteria is inhibited due to nutritional deficiency. As we have seen, when the lactobacteria are not thriving and do not constitute a large percentage of the colon population, the colon becomes prey to gas-forming and other harmful types of microorganisms.

Science now recognizes that the specific role of lactose is to provide food for the healthy colon flora. Lactose is the only carbohydrate to reach the colon in large amounts because of its slow absorption factor.[13] Thus, it will reach the colon to feed the flora.

Nature always has a reason for its often mysterious ways.

Fructooligosaccharide (FOS)

Fructooligosaccharides (FOS) is one of the products claimed to benefit the colon B. *bifidum*. In nature, this natural sugar is found in Jerusalem artichokes, onions, burdock, and rye. It is obtained commercially by the action of fructosyltransferase on sucrose (white table sugar). Organically grown Jerusalem artichoke powder, which contains naturally occurring FOS, is one of the products on the market at this time from a natural source.

Some *Bifidobacteria* do utilize FOS as a carbohydrate source, but so do some harmful types of bacteria, such as *Klebsiella pneumonia*. However, B. *bifidum* specifically does not utilize FOS as a food source.[14]

L. *acidophilus* and B. *bifidum* are perhaps the most important bacterial constituents in the healthy adult human colon. Their primary need is for the milk sugar, lactose, found most amply in whey. Theoretically, once the pathogens are removed, FOS would be helpful as an alternative to whey for those who are lactose intolerant.

Maltose and Dextrin

Maltose and dextrin are carbohydrates that can be metabolized by the colon lactobacteria. Maltose is a carbohydrate found in malt, which is germinated from whole grains. Dextrin is formed in the digestive tract as a result of digesting complex carbohydrates, including whole grains. A study done by the FDA found dextrin to also be effective in colonizing the intestine without use of oral lactobacteria.[15]

This is one reason why a diet high in natural whole grains and complex carbohydrates is so beneficial to health. Lactose in whey exerts the strongest dietary influence in transforming the colon flora to one predominated by lactobacteria. Maltose and dextrose are important secondary foods that promote a strong, positive influence on beneficial colon lactobacteria.[16]

CHAPTER 18

Golden Grains

In addition to sweet dairy whey, the most important food to support a healthy colon flora is whole grains, ground fresh, at home, right before cooking. Grains prepared in this manner have a high content of nutrients that are easily assimilated into the body. Eating freshly ground, freshly cooked grains will give you more energy and a higher quality of sustained energy.

The Chinese character for "chi" (loosely translated as "energy" or "life force") includes the central image of steam rising up from a bowl of cereal grains. The body requires large amounts of complex carbohydrates (grains and vegetables) to constantly provide us with the lasting energy we need daily to sustain us. Whole grains are the very best source of complex carbohydrates when bought and freshly ground before cooking to release their full nutritional value and chi. "Cereal-in-a-box" cannot provide these benefits.

Do you recognize this scenario? At 7 o'clock Monday morning, you eat a bowl of hot oatmeal for breakfast and feel hungry within an hour. Tuesday morning at 7 o'clock, you decide to try eating two scrambled eggs, toast, and coffee. But again, you are hungry one hour after your meal. So, at 7 o'clock Wednesday morning, you gobble hot cakes, butter, and milk for breakfast. Oh no, hungry again within an hour after breakfast! Why do you get hungry again so soon after breakfast every day?

Oh well, you have to get to work. You can gulp down a cup of coffee or two at 10 AM. You can only hope that the caffeine from the coffee will hold you over until noon, when you can grab a hamburger. That double-decker burger goes down easily, and all is well until 2 PM. But that hungry feeling surfaces again. Another burger would be great; better grab another cup of coffee to make it until dinner.

Stop here! This routine is not creating sustaining energy, it is drain-ing the adrenal glands. Adrenaline is for "flight or fight," not for work. Furthermore, this pattern of frequent eating and caffeine consump-tion can cause hypoglycemia. If we want to sustain energy, we must consume adequate amounts of glycogen, which is found in fresh, unoxidized grains. Only then will this scenario of short-lived satia-tion cease.

Adrenal Glands and Glycogen

The adrenal glands, which sit on top of the kidneys, have both saved our lives and, in some cases, taken our lives. Adrenaline, pro-duced in the adrenal glands, stimulates the flight-or-fight response when an extra amount of quick, temporary energy is needed. This response was very useful for humans living in the jungle who needed to react to sudden threats by hungry predators.

Today, after millions of years of evolution, it appears that at least some people in industrial societies may be using adrenaline for gen-eral activity because of the glycogen deficiency in their diet.

This glycogen deficiency is due to consuming the wrong types of carbohydrates. Contrary to popular belief, all carbohydrates are not equal. There is quite a difference between simple carbohydrates and complex carbohydrates and how they are utilized by the human body.

Simple carbohydrates, sugars in their simplest form, can be used for metabolism of energy. In terms of food, this includes donuts, cakes, cookies, candies, and sugar. We tend to eat these foods for snacks, quick energy boosts, and, all too often, as meal substitutes. These simple sugars are metabolized quickly by the body. With sucrose or table sugar, there is often a quick rise in blood sugar level, followed by an dramatic drop. This drop gives rise to hunger, feelings of hy-poglycemia, and other symptoms.

Complex carbohydrates are just that. Chemically, they are combi-nations of simple sugars that form more complex substances. These are carbohydrates in the forms made by nature, such as potatoes, vegetables, squashes, and cereal grains. When these foods are eaten, they take time to digest and are released into the bloodstream slowly. This provides a more stable release of food that the body can metabolize into energy over a longer period of time.

Refined grains and refined, packaged cereal products do not have the same effect as freshly-ground grains. This is because most of the nutrients in refined cereal and grain products are lost due to oxidation and long shelf life. Thus, many manufacturers add nutrients back into their devitalized products.

The lack of sustained glycogen drives the body to demand more carbohydrates at times during the day when there is energy depletion. Craving for snacks is a signal that the body needs more glycogen. Due to eating poor-quality carbohydrates, many people have depleted their store of energy and are running on snacks and adrenal energy, which depletes their body even further.

Carbohydrates are broken down by the body into glucose, the most important carbohydrate in body metabolism. Only so much glucose can circulate in the bloodstream at any given time. Ideally, there is an excess of glucose, which is converted to glycogen and stored in the liver and skeletal muscles. As more glucose is needed, the body can draw on this stored glycogen and can convert it back into glucose. Oxygen and glucose are necessary to prevent fatigue from constant physical exertion.[1]

In my estimation, many people suffer from a lack of energy due to a deficiency of the stored glycogen that is meant to be used as our true energy source. Adrenaline will be available, if needed, in an emergency only.[2]

A steady intake of a diet low in naturally occurring, fresh, complex carbohydrates and high in snack foods, simple sugars, and refined carbohydrates can cause many of the social problems we see in our society. The human system is on stress alert in the absence of an emergency.

There is a great deal of research linking low blood sugar (hypoglycemia) to criminal and antisocial behavior.[3,4] Glycogen deficiency can cause stress, nervousness, violent behavior, irrational thoughts, depression and, if carried to the extreme, aggressive physical confrontations. Under stress, the adrenal glands begin to produce hormones at an accelerated rate. The motor is running on the wrong fuel while the driver is getting mixed signals and could lose control.

Whole Grains for Energy

Many answers can be found as we return to simplicity. Recall the television photos of African tribal women using a mortar and pestle to grind fresh, dry grains. It is no coincidence that one of the best sources of glycogen is found in these unoxidized grains. Grains contain cellulose on the outer surface that seals nutrients inside the seed. In the grinding process, the cellulose outer coat of the grain is broken. When the ground grain is immediately placed in a container of water and cooked to become a thick, hot cereal, all the essential nutrients are trapped and are able to provide five hours of sustaining energy.

For thousands of years, people in all parts of the world have been eating grains prepared by this method. These people are able to work long and hard. They are sustained by the glycogen stores in their liver that drip as glucose into their bloodstream. This process takes us back prior to cereal-in-a-box and gives us lasting energy for the day's activities.

This experience of sustained energy need not be limited to tribal peoples in developing countries. In modern society, there is a basic nutritional deficiency of glycogen in the food chain that is not being addressed. When grains are prepared as above, this deficiency is eliminated. By following the simple, natural, and satisfying routine of milling dry grains for at least one meal a day, we experience more sustaining energy at a deeper level. We are also likely to lose extra weight and keep it off.

I have seen the health of entire families restored for the better when the needed glycogen is replaced. Just try a bowl of cereal prepared properly, and you will see results.

Grains should be purchased in their whole-seed form, with only the outer husk removed. They should be kept refrigerated until used to prevent spoilage of the natural oils and oxidation of other nutrients. Once a grain is rolled, cracked, ground, or milled into flour, it

BREAKFAST RECIPE

Grind your grains for fast cooking, easy preparation, freshly ground flavor, and high energy that lasts. This recipe takes about 20 minutes to prepare.

Grind dry, whole grains in an electric blender at a high speed to desired fineness.

Add 1/3 cup ground long-grain brown rice to 2 cups cold water OR Add 1/3 cup ground whole oats to 1 cup cold water.

Bring to a boil at high heat, stirring frequently. Turn heat down to low. Cover and simmer for 15 minutes. Turn off heat, let stand covered for 5 more minutes.

Serve cereal in a bowl. Cover with desired amount of liquid whey.

Makes 1 serving

BREAKFAST FOR YOU AND YOUR LACTOBACTERIA

Mix 2 to 3 tablespoons of sweet whey in a glass of water. Just before eating, pour whey drink over your cereal.

If you like, add a pinch of cinnamon and a little honey or maple syrup.

GOLDEN PANCAKES

1 cup water mixed with 3 to 5 tablespoons whey
1 egg, slightly beaten
1/2 cup freshly ground pastry wheat flour
1/2 cup freshly ground oat flour
1 teaspoon cinnamon
1 tablespoon baking powder, aluminum-free
1 pinch sea salt

Grind whole pastry wheat and whole hulled oats in the blender to a fine-consistency flour. Sift dry ingredients into a bowl.

Alternately add eggs and whey liquid to the dry ingredients, gently mixing together. Let mixture stand for a few minutes while the griddle heats up. Cook pancakes on the griddle and turn when golden brown.

Makes 2 servings.

can become rancid and lose most of its nutritional value. The fresher the grain is and the closer to its natural state, the more nutrients are retained. When freshly ground at home and cooked immediately, grains retain essential nutrients for our health. Refined, oxidized grains with added vitamins are not what nature intended for our total health.

Grains can be used two to three meals a day, are delicious, and can be cooked in a variety of ways. The preparation of whole grains is limited only by the imagination. They can be cooked whole, ground coarse, or fine ground to give assorted textures. When very finely ground, they can be used as flour in recipes.

You can combine different grains to give a variety of flavors and energetic qualities. Oat berries combined with long-grain brown rice make an excellent breakfast cereal combination. Try adding some wild rice for a different flavor.

Other nutritious whole grains include triticale, short-grain brown rice, sweet rice, basmati rice, millet, barley, rye, and buckwheat. Amaranth, kamut and quinoa are more exotic grains worth trying, as they are also very tasty. Of course, avoid any grain you don't like or that doesn't agree with you.

These delicious cereals provide real nourishment for our bodies, giving us true energy and bountiful fresh nutrients. Grains eaten with whey give bulk to the colon and provide the colon lactobacteria flora with lactose and other nutrients necessary for their growth naturally. This is the perfect start for a busy day.

Fiber - Just Passing Through

Everyone asks about fiber. Fiber is the indigestible part of carbohydrates, often called roughage. Passing through the digestive tract, fiber reaches the colon, where different types of fiber have different actions.

There are two main types of fiber, "insoluble" and "soluble." Soluble fiber is found in fruits, legumes, and grains such as oats. The primary action of soluble fiber is to delay the emptying time of the stomach (so does adding a little oil or butter to your grains before eating them), which is helpful in regulating blood sugar. Soluble fiber is especially noted for its action in helping lower cholesterol in the body.

Insoluble fiber, as found in natural balance in vegetables and whole grains, is considered the type most beneficial to the colon. Insoluble fiber acts as an intestinal broom, gives bulk and softness to the stool, and assists the movement of feces through the colon. This movement of bulk slightly stretches the muscular colon wall, helping to maintain its good muscle tone.

The body needs both, but you do not need to ingest fiber supplements, psyllium, or bran to get fiber: it's already in our food! In fact, it is my experience that most people use too many fiber supplements, creating more problems than they solve. All the fiber in the world will not help unless we have the correct colon flora.

CHAPTER 19

Fasting and Other Food Follies

The following foods are those that, from my experience, cause the most colon problems. There may be other foods that cause problems for an individual, according to his or her constitution or tolerance. The foods I am presenting here, across the board, are harmful to the acidophilus colon flora.

Dry Foods and Fiber

All dry foods tend to clog the colon and cause a myriad of problems. These foods include breads, bagels, dried fruits, and foods eaten in a powdered form without liquids added, such as green algae tablets or powders, dry fiber bars, and the like. This list also includes dry granola cereals and bran products.

Dehydrated food has had the water removed from it for convenient storage and extension of shelf life. Foods are not meant to be eaten in this form. They must be rehydrated before eating. This means, simply, that dried fruits can be softened in water overnight. Dry nutritional or algae powders should always be reconstituted in water before they are ingested.

Breads are not dehydrated, but too much bread tends to keep the colon contents hard and dry. You will not crave bread if you increase your intake of the glycogen your body needs with freshly ground, cooked grains.

When we ingest foods that lack sufficient water content, our own body fluids will have to compensate for the deficiency. Excess consumption of dry, hard foods is a major cause of constipation.

Fiber is an essential part of the diet, best consumed in its natural form, as found in fruits and vegetables, which have a high water content. Fiber products, isolated from whole foods, cause more problems than they solve. Combining incorrect types of fiber with a deficient colon flora interferes with normal elimination and actually makes for worse elimination problems. Get fiber in the forms made by nature: fresh fruits, vegetables, and whole grains cooked in water.

Popcorn

Popcorn is the king of dry foods. Its reputation as being a good source of fiber is a myth. Perhaps eating popcorn in moderation can be tolerated, but I have seen popcorn eaters who have terrible blockages in their colons. The outer husk of the popcorn kernel (the pieces that get caught in the teeth) is indigestible, hard, heat-treated cellulose. As an alternative to eating popcorn, I recommend a tasty rice product that is found in health food stores. Although the product looks and tastes like popcorn, it is completely free of kernels.

Alcohol

I am obliged to mention this product because it is so commonly used in our society. My clients often inquire about what effects drinking alcohol may have on their colon. I can only emphasize the point that alcohol must be used in moderation. Alcohol destroys the lactobacteria in the colon. When clients ingest any kind of alcohol, the initial growth of the lactobacteria implant fails. To achieve a balanced immune system, forget alcohol instead of forgetting your health.

High-Protein, High-Fat Diets

Research shows that the main contributors to colon cancer around the world are diets high in fat and diets high in protein. Populations eating diets high in whole grains and vegetables, low in protein and fats, have a much lower incidence of colon cancer, diabetes, and heart disease. These conditions rapidly increase with industrialization and are most prevalent in developed Western nations. The studies also show that high protein diets combined with high fat intake cause harmful bacteria to proliferate in the colon and create toxic by-products.[1,2,3,4]

In particular, too much red meat causes problems. Animal products are best consumed in moderation. Eating meat two to three times a day is massive overconsumption. Red meats should be eaten only occasionally and in small amounts. Fish, fowl, and eggs are excellent sources of animal protein if they are raised naturally, without use of hormones and antibiotics.

Everyone today is concerned about fat. The problem is both the type and the quantity of fats we are eating. Steam or gently stir-fry foods instead of deep frying. Use high-quality oils, such as olive or sesame, that have been cold pressed without the use of heat or chemicals.[5,6,7]

Raw Foods

Consuming raw fish from any location is really asking for trouble. Without a microscope, we are unable to see the parasites residing in raw fish and are unaware of their presence. Since these parasites are destroyed at normal cooking temperatures, the solution seems obvious.

Some people eat raw eggs regularly, and many of them get salmonella poisoning. The Centers for Disease Control report salmonellosis is increasing.

As the hazards from consuming raw dairy products today are high, use only pasteurized milk. In our industrialized society, where we do not personally care for the cow's hygiene, infection from a multi-resistant microorganism (such as *Salmonella*) is possible. The possible risks and benefits should be considered.

Gas-Forming Foods

Very often, raw vegetables cause intestinal gas in people. Broccoli, cabbage, and cauliflower are particular problems for some individuals. Beans of all types are well known for causing flatulence, but any food that doesn't digest well will cause problems in the colon. Use common sense. If any food gives you gas, don't eat it. If a food doesn't agree with you, you will not assimilate it properly.

Fasting and Detoxification: Use Caution

Many people understand the term "detox" to be either the process of drug detoxification or as defined by *Alcoholics Anonymous*. But detox, short for "detoxification," is a general term for the process whereby a system rids itself of toxins.

There are health-seeking individuals who believe that they need to detoxify their bodies from a lifetime of exposure to pollution, pesticides, and harmful foods. These people often turn to the age-old treatment of fasting to accomplish this goal. However, there are several caveats to this approach. Fasting is no longer as appropriate as it once was.

This true story of a 55-year-old client illustrates several reasons why fasting can be inappropriate. My client's livelihood required that he work in close proximity to harmful chemicals. On his own, this man decided he would benefit from a strict cleansing fast.

He began his regimen by consuming only water for a few days. The following week, he drank only juice. He did well until the tenth day, when he began to feel weak. He called a nutritionist for advice, who correctly instructed him to start eating soft foods, such as cooked vegetables, for nourishment and in order to slow the detoxification process. Although he followed this advice, he became weaker.

The nutritionist suspected that chemicals from his occupational exposure had been stored in his tissues and, due to the fast, were being released into his bloodstream. Within 10 more days, he became nervous, his speech was slurred, and his muscles began to cramp and stiffen. Yet he continued this self-imposed, radical cleansing routine for two months, without ever consulting a health professional again.

At this time, he modified his routine to include much bed rest, a strict nutritious food intake, and light exercise. At the end of a year and a half, he gradually started to return to normal.

When an individual undertakes radical detoxification without understanding the mechanisms that adversely affect health, the results may be worse than doing nothing at all. In this example, the man threw his balance off completely by detoxifying too quickly. The toxins latent in his system were not noticeable prior to the strict fast since his system, compensating at its best level, was in homeostasis.

Fasting releases toxins stored in the body. In many people, the liver cannot keep pace with this increased burden and is unable to deal with the released toxins effectively. The toxins are then thrown into the blood circulation. This is why a person can experience severe symptoms, as did this man.[8]

When chemicals and drugs stored in the tissues are dumped into the bloodstream, a person will very often re-experience their effects. Since a variety of chemicals may be released at the same time, the effects are unpredictable and may cause great damage. Our bodies are not meant to handle so many toxins all at once, let alone in the weakened, fasting state.

Fasting was a much more straightforward process in simpler days. Historically, nature cure doctors used fasting, fruits, vegetables, and other cures drawn from nature to treat their clients. These doctors would fast clients for as many as 40 to 100 days. Leon Chaitow, a prominent naturopath and osteopath in England, states this cannot be done anymore. He says,

> If we put somebody on a long fast who's had steroids, antibiotics, or fifteen other strong drugs, God knows what's in their fatty tissues and what will come flooding back into the system... We can't expect the same results anymore. We've changed the organism so we must modify the approach.[9]

In this day and age, with widespread use of drugs of all types, pesticides, and other chemicals in the food chain, the human system is being challenged as never before in history. When someone goes on an extended fast, all these things will suddenly dump into the bloodstream, causing immense discomfort and possibly overloading the system's capacity. Prolonged or excessive fasting throws more toxins into a situation that is already toxic. Continual fasting and cleansing further weaken the system, leaving it vulnerable to illness or pathogens.

Leading health professionals no longer recommend extended fasts.[10,11] Experts state that fasts of a few days at a time are the longest that should be undertaken. If a fast longer than this is indicated, it is best done under supervision of a qualified professional with experience in this area.

I have found fasting to be unnecessary in almost all cases. There is certainly no need for detoxifying the body to be a dramatic or traumatic event, as it often has been in the old-school tradition of long-term, radical fasts. Do not experiment with your health. It is not worth it.

Toxins that have accumulated over a lifetime cannot be eliminated in a day, a week, or even a month. The general guideline health professionals use is that it will take one month for each year of life to effect a change. In fact, it often takes much longer, depending on the person, his or her constitution, and circumstances.

Alternative approaches that cleanse the body without fasting are available. Licensed acupuncturists, well trained in Chinese herbal medicine, can skillfully adjust the interplay between cleansing and nourishing an individual. The ancient Chinese medicine practitioners understood the necessity of clearing toxins and pathogens out of the body.

However, an overwhelming amount of toxins released into circulation suppresses the immune system, and toxins are not effectively excreted. When the toxins are powerful and the person is deficient or weak, the primary consideration in Chinese medicine is to build up the strength and immunity of the individual. Cleansing is inappropriate and will only further weaken the person, putting at risk their chance for full recovery of health.

Modern research confirms that an undernourished, depleted person is less able to eliminate certain toxins. With proper nourishment comes improved excretion of toxins.[12,13] The good health and stamina of a person is what keeps them from being overwhelmed by any toxins or pathogens. A person can be cleared of toxins at their own pace and avoid undergoing a cleansing regimen that can be dramatic and possibly traumatic.

The colon must be addressed in any detoxification program. When toxins are being cleared from the system, whether due to fasting, herbal treatment, or the natural processes of the body, elimination must be facilitated. The normal routes are through the skin, in the form of sweat, and through the urine and feces.

As a greater than usual amount of toxins will pass through the colon, this may cause adverse changes in an already damaged colon flora. For example, when people have their mercury fillings removed, traces of the fillings pass through the gastrointestinal tract (unless precautions are taken) or mercury vapors may pass into the system, damaging the colon flora.[14]

When properly nourished and optimally functioning, the body can follow its own natural wisdom about how and when to eliminate any toxins. Like a good housekeeper, it knows the best time to do light cleaning or heavy cleaning. The body loses this wisdom when overwhelmed with pollution, from within or without, but regains it with assistance and fine tuning.

The wisdom of the body is enhanced once the slightly acid colon flora is established. We have to offer our bodies a solid foundation from which to work.

The law of purification reigns in nature. In winter, the tops of mountains are covered with snow. In spring, snow melts, rapid water flows downriver. River banks rise, clearing debris and stagnant ponds. If we follow the laws of Mother Nature and keep ourselves clear of pollution as much as possible, we shall survive in health.

CHAPTER 20

Nutrition, Lifestyle, and Colon Health

Although this is not a book about nutrition, I must directly address the topic of diet, because clients are constantly bringing this issue to my attention. I see people who are experiencing toxicity not only from an unhealthy colon, but also from consuming an excess of the wrong foods. Eventually, the combination of a toxic colon and deficient diet culminates in illness and fatigue.

Reaching this point, people think they need some sort of supplement or herb in order to resolve their various ailments. Taking a shotgun approach, they overwhelm the system, consuming multitudes of natural and synthetic supplements from their ever-expanding home pharmacy, hoping something will hit the right place, and all will be well again.

But they are still sick and tired. The shotgun approach is similar to flooding the carburetor in a car. The body is unable to metabolize supplements taken in excess. Too much is as bad as too little. We need to take a step back, set aside the supplements, and assess the person's status.

First, the colon needs to be addressed. A balanced diet and lifestyle need to be followed for lasting results. Then any remaining health concerns can be taken care of appropriately.

Nature did not intend nutrition to be confusing, yet many people are so confused they have lost the basic knowledge of what to eat!

Our confusion regarding how to provide fuel for our bodily functions has paralleled the industrialization of society. Even many health-conscious individuals, willing to take responsibility for their own health, are unable to identify appropriate guidelines.

As we approach nutrition, let us return to simplicity. What we eat most determines our basic health. Make the shift gradually, slowly substituting natural foods for junk foods until natural foods are dominant in the diet. For example, if you love chocolate, eat some chocolate, just eat less. Eventually, you can use cocoa powder and a natural sweetener to satisfy your craving while simultaneously avoiding the refined sugar in chocolate.

A Balanced Diet

In order to achieve and maintain maximum health, grains and whey should constitute a regular part of a well-balanced diet that includes a variety of good-quality foods. An ideal balanced diet for most people is 70% to 80% complex carbohydrates, including vegetables and fruits, 15% protein, and about 15% natural fats. This diet meets daily requirements.

Quality for Life

Quality refers to aspects of food that cannot be measured, such as how fresh food is, how it is grown, and how long it is stored. These are very significant considerations.

Much more than just so many units of nutrients, food imparts life force or vitality to us. However, only fresh food can impart this quality of life force or living energy. Modern science realizes that nutrients and enzymes are more abundant in fresh foods than in old foods. Storage, manufacturing, or shipping procedures can likewise compromise the nutrient capacity and life force present in foods.

We were not meant to live on a diet consisting of canned, processed, and frozen foods. These types of food may contain some nutrients but have little or no life force and have lost most of their enzymes. They should constitute only a very small part of your diet, if any part at all.

Unfortunately, awareness of the importance of organically grown foods, both vegetable and animal, is growing all too slowly. Pesticides can overload the liver and the body with toxins. No studies have ever been done on the cumulative effect of pesticides in the human body or on the interaction of the many different kinds of pesticides within the human body.

Most animals are not raised under ideal conditions. Cattle may be eating pesticide-sprayed grass and feed. Animals are fed hormones to increase their growth rate and are given antibiotics to fend off the incidence of disease. Due to the prevalence of polluted water, fish may contain chemicals and heavy metals. The larger the body of the fish, the greater the accumulation of contaminants. These substances are passed through the food chain to humans.

One of the culprits in the current overuse of antibiotics is the widespread occurrence of antibiotics in our diets, due to their abundant use in raising livestock and fish. This use results in trace amounts of antibiotics in meat products and commercially raised fish. Even minute amounts have a cumulative effect when these foods are consumed daily and in combination.

Many vegetables, herbs, and fruits can be grown in our own backyards. Health food stores usually carry a selection of fresh, organic produce. Some also carry organic, range-fed, hormone-free animal products. Even supermarkets are beginning to carry a small supply of organic produce for their customers. Ask your grocers.

Quality Water

Good, pure water is essential for all the cells and tissues in our bodies and, thus, for our health. Unfortunately, hundreds of chemicals are now present in our drinking water, unseen by the naked eye.

The Environmental Protection Agency (EPA) claims that 800 water systems, serving 30 million people, have excessive levels of lead in their drinking water. The effects of lead in the human system range from miscarriages, infants with low birth weight, and central nervous system disorders in the young. Adults are at risk for high blood pressure and kidney disease.[1] The presence of lead is only one example of the many problems with the drinking water in America. In order to avoid consuming these chemicals, we must purify our water.

Many different types of units are available, but all are not equally effective in removing impurities. Any purification unit used should be tested by an independent source in order to confirm its effectiveness. Verify that the product has been tested and certified by the National Sanitation Foundation (NSF), which is one such foundation for independent testing and information.

A 0.5-micron pore size is necessary to filter out *Giardia lamblia* and *Cryptosporidium*, waterborne parasites that are found in some water supplies. Despite methods used in water purification plants, there have been many outbreaks of these organisms. These conditions have been widely reported in *Newsweek, The Wall Street Journal,* and other publications throughout the last several years. In 1993, *Infectious Disease News* reported that 281,000 people in Milwaukee were infected by *Cryptosporidium* in the city's water supply.[2]

For providing pure drinking water, machine dispensers and bottled water are not as cost-effective as owning a home filter system. In recent years, many improved purification units have appeared on the market, so the consumer will need to do a little research before investing in a water purifier.

Some individuals find reverse-osmosis systems to produce satisfactory water. I prefer a solid carbon-block filter system that retains the naturally occurring minerals in water. Although distilled water is sometimes useful during a detoxification program, nature does not produce distilled water. We need the mineral components found in naturally clean water.

Assimilation

It's not only what we eat that's important, it's what we assimilate. If food is not digested properly, it will arrive at the colon undigested, and this can lead to colon problems.

To maximize assimilation of micronutrients in the upper digestive tract, a supplement of a small amount of plant-derived enzymes that contain amylase, protease, lipase, and cellulase can be used as a dietary supplement. Amylase assists carbohydrate digestion, protease assists protein digestion, and lipase improves digestion of fats. Cellulase specifically helps digestion of the fibrous matter in vegetables and fruits. Even though small quantities of enzymes do exist in foods, a small amount of enzymes is an easy way to boost our own digestive powers.

Edward Howell, biochemist and nutrition researcher, was the first to recognize and describe the role of food enzymes in human nutrition. He developed enzymes that would compensate for the deficiencies in the human food chain. Dr. Howell's book, *Enzyme Nutrition*, is the culmination of 20 years of study. It is an abridged form of his original 700-page book, which contained over 700 references.[3]

Warm Foods for Warm Bodies

When we eat, our bodies warm the food to body temperature in order to digest it. That is one reason why too many cold, raw foods deplete our digestive functioning. Many individuals experience indigestion and gas from eating raw foods. Most people do best with about 80% to 90% cooked foods and 10% to 20% raw vegetables and fruits. This varies seasonally and according to the person. In the cold of winter, anyone with common sense will eat very few, if any, raw, cold foods.

Cooking makes many nutrients available for assimilation by the body, such as the B vitamins in string beans. Gently steaming vegetables with small amounts of water conserves the most nutrients.

Eating uncooked grains, no matter how long they are soaked, places a great strain on the digestive tract and can cause congestion in the colon. Warm foods help nourish us at all levels and keep us warm, happy people in warm, healthy bodies.

Yogurt

Yogurt is an ancient food that has been consumed by nomadic tribes around the world. The tribes made yogurt by transforming the milk of their herds with live starter cultures of bacteria. Yogurt cultures were prized, passed down from generation to generation, and shared among families. The source of their starter culture was, and still is, from one or more of their milk-producing animals, whether cows, sheep, camels, horses, or other milk-producing animals. The cultures were live and very strong. Today's commercial yogurt is very weak by comparison, and many of the cultures used are not ideal. Bovine-source lactobacteria are used commercially to transform milk into yogurt, and most companies pasteurize the yogurt after the culture has been added.

For the best-quality yogurt, look for brands that use *Lactobacillus acidophilus* and *Bifidobacterium bifidum*. The label should specifically state that the cultures were added after pasteurization. This type of yogurt will help maintain the colon flora, especially with the addition of high-grade sweet whey.

Acidophilus milk and yogurt are popular, nutritious, and delicious foods. They will not, however, transform the colon flora into a beneficial flora for many of the same reasons discussed in earlier chapters. Studies show that both yogurt and acidophilus milk are useful health products, but one should not count on them to replenish a depleted colon flora.

YOGURT SHAKE

Add 5 tablespoons yogurt

to 1 cup water or milk.

Add 1 to 2 tablespoons of sweet whey.

Add sweetener or other ingredients,

such as fruit, if desired.

Blend to the consistency of a milkshake.

Exercise as a Way of Life

Our forefathers and mothers did not have to plan an exercise routine. They were busy, active people, chopping wood, hauling water, planting and harvesting crops, hunting for food, and socializing.

Life is movement. In these times, when most of our movement seems to be intellectual, it is important to remember to move and enjoy our body's movements as well. Movement and activity are essential parts of health and life, influencing our physical, mental, emotional, and spiritual well-being.

When aerobic activities are adapted to an appropriate level for an individual's health and age, overall fitness can be maintained. Aerobic movements are those that increase the heartbeat to a certain rate above resting. These activities include walking, running, trampoline bouncing, swimming, and cycling.

Just as the air around us is in motion, so is the lymphatic system around our cells. Our cells function better with a clean lymphatic system. A colon that is clean and free of putrefaction improves both the lymphatic system and overall health. Two main areas of the body act as pumps to move the lymphatic system. The lymph fluids will not move on their own, but require the action of these pumps, through exercise, to keep them moving healthily. These areas are the movements of the calves and, most importantly, the movements of the rib cage. With good exercise, we move our legs (calves) and breathe deeply, which moves the rib cage. For the average person, exercising three days a week will keep the lymphatic system in shape. In my experience, individuals who exercise regularly have good muscle tone in their colon and enhanced elimination.

Squat for Health

Sitting on the toilet with legs at a right angle, feet on the floor, causes unnecessary pressure on the colon, which can lead to hemorrhoids and longer transit time. This position contributes to straining at the toilet and eventual constipation.

Human beings are designed by nature to eliminate in a squatting

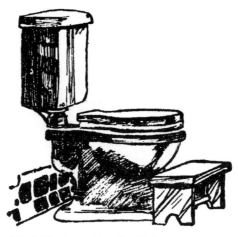

Figure 10. A Footstool by the Toilet Aids Elimination

position. A small footstool, about 6 inches up to 14 inches in height, can be very helpful to aid the colon during elimination. Place the stool under your feet while sitting on the toilet. This sets the body in a comfortable squatting position, allowing the colon to be more relaxed and removing pressure from the hemorrhoidal veins. Using the footstool can help prevent hemorrhoids and promote easier elimination.

Meditation and Relaxation

Meditation is popular and it seems appropriate to say a few words about this subject as it is connected to total health. When the colon is normal and free of toxins, the bloodstream is clean, the nervous system is not irritated with impurities, meditation is easier, and thoughts are clearer.

Electroencephalography, or EEG, is a high-tech method to measure the electrical energy generated by nerve cells in the brain. With EEG, at least four levels of human brain waves have been classified according to frequency in cycles per second, which is measured in hertz (Hz). The deepest level of frequency is "delta," unconscious, deep sleep. "Theta" is the next level, in the range of 4 to 8 Hz of activity. Only a few people, such as long-term meditators and yogis, are conscious at this frequency level.[4] The next level is "alpha," in the range of 8 to 14 Hz, a relaxed, artistic, intuitive, creative level. Alpha activity disappears with visual attention in most people. Fourth is the waking state, "beta."[5] Beta activity is above 14 Hz and is associated with mental activity, occurring in bursts in the anterior part of the brain.[6]

Meditation techniques begin at beta, the waking frequency level, with a goal to reach and stay in alpha, the creative level, as long as desired, to observe your own thoughts. Rather than starting at beta, it is much easier to stay in alpha while in the process of awaking from delta (deep sleep) to the next level, theta (semi-deep sleep). To be in alpha, awake consciously without opening your eyes. As soon as the eyes open, beta frequency and daily activity start once more.

It takes a few attempts each morning to become consciously aware to keep the eyes closed. Hold them shut for as long as you wish. After a few days, you will be able to stay in alpha when awakening, before arising. Once in alpha, it is simple to observe your thoughts and "clear the tape," so to speak, of unnecessary chatter that clogs the mind in the waking state of beta.

Once cleared, the mind literally relaxes. On that clear level, we can achieve new human potential to make this planet a better, more harmonious, conscious planet to live on collectively, without an overload of stress. Nature's time is slower than societal time. As below, so above.

Enjoy Life!

Consider the foods you eat. Be aware of their effect on you, your energy level, your moods, and feeling of well-being. Notice which foods are digested easily. Do you feel satisfied after eating? Experiment with new foods. Find and eat foods you enjoy, that impart sustained energy, a sense of well-being, and enable you to achieve your goals in life.

You should not have to spend much time thinking about your diet. Once you're in good health, with your body in balance, it is easier to recognize both your basic and changing needs. Your cravings will become healthier. You will want to move and exercise.

Being in balance allows us to live our life with awareness of how to fulfill our needs simply in a harmonious way. You need to listen to yourself. Experiment, find out what works for you. Once you are on the right track, forget about it and enjoy your life!

CHAPTER 21

Achieve Maximum Health

Today, an ounce of prevention is worth much more than a pound of cure! Numerous researchers are currently trying to find cures for diseases of all kinds. Billions of dollars and years of dedication are being spent in this pursuit.

It is ironic that the cost for treating disease continues to soar even while true prevention is available. If people want to achieve health, the solution is no longer a mystery. Unnecessary suffering can be eliminated. True prevention means being as healthy as possible. This, ultimately, is the only solution that can potentially save trillions of dollars in health care costs. To do that, we must have basic knowledge of how life works from the foundation up, or it is a house built on sand.

When people are born without knowledge and live in a high-tech environment, they must be guided to stay well. Animals living in nature do not have such deficiencies in education. They learn the laws of nature from the day of their birth. The young learn to respect themselves, others, and the laws of nature in a very short time or they die. Just because we have created a technological lifestyle does not mean we can get away from the basic laws of nature.

More than 50 years of industrialization have made a radical impact on our health and environment. If we do not take steps to return to basics as much as possible through natural nutrition and lifestyle, we will perpetuate the very imbalances we have created due to the ignorance of our past.

Yes, we are subject to the laws of cause and effect, and we will be until the end of time. The choice is ours for a while longer. To make up for lost time, every conscious person on this planet needs to pitch in by educating those who are in the dark. This can be accomplished when we become responsible about our lives and the lives of those around us.

Education at the grammar school level should include good, sensible toilet training, basic hygiene, and nutrition. This type of education would be a giant step toward eliminating future sickness and ignorance. When the first generation of school children educated in this manner become parents, they will comprise an educated public, and health will not be the issue it is at present.

Ideally, centers for the total art of healing would include every safe, effective approach that can be made available. We can appropriately use all methods that are scientifically based. Eastern and Western medical traditions combined will make powerful medicine that offers a truly comprehensive approach to wellness if the population really desires a healthy, happy life. A few such centers are starting to open.

This is the intelligent approach to survival in the 21st century and beyond. We are at the crossroads, and time will see if the ego can step aside and let truth in. We must live in harmony with one another and with nature to survive into the future.

By using our intelligence and common sense and by following natural laws with tried-and-true scientific examples, we can eliminate most unnecessary suffering on this planet and start enjoying life! The bacteria have been here for billions of years, long before humans arrived on earth. One bacteria can create approximately 17 million offspring every 24 hours.[1] They have unique inherent intelligence and mechanisms for adjusting to any new environmental situation with which they are confronted. Antibiotic resistance is only one example.[2] Microorganisms have already started to outsmart human beings, as we have seen.

Why is *Mycobacterium tuberculosis* back with a vengeance? As of this writing, all of the antibiotics in the arsenal are becoming ineffective against tuberculosis. Yet tuberculosis was thought to be conquered only a few decades ago. This is only one result of the immunity of microorganisms becoming stronger than ours.

Because of many recent ecological changes, no one, at present, can predict the direction of the evolving microcosm. However, any intelligent person can look at the past, apply the facts to the future, and grasp the potential.

Microorganisms are not intentionally trying to harm the human body. They are adjusting to a shift from their normal balance imposed on them by industrialization. Recovering from this shift may be too great a task for the human body without immediate support. The result can be a weakened immune system that is passed on to future generations, eroding the constitution of the family tree.

In just 50 years, our nation's health has been radically changed. Those who are now 40 years old and younger are manifesting successively weaker immune systems, with higher incidence of chronic, immune, and fatigue disorders than the older generation that was raised on wholesome food prior to widespread use of antibiotics and environmental contaminants.

We cannot keep on a mission of search and destroy. We must normalize the colon flora pH to eliminate harmful microorganisms and to replenish our natural protective shield. Lactobacteria act as a protective shield, preventing disease and reinforcing a strong immune system.

The first step any good gardener takes is to eliminate pests by upgrading the quality of the soil, which improves the health of the plants. A healthy, slightly acidic colon is the soil of the body. By reestablishing the normal colon flora and maintaining its viability, health and longevity can be promoted from within.

There are many approaches to the resolution of human body imbalances. In all cases, the colon is the foundation. Webster Implant Technique provides an answer to the lost colon flora. At birth we are supported by breast milk, receiving our first lactobacteria implant. When the first implant is destroyed, the natural course is to receive a second lactobacteria implant as an adult. The implant must then be provided with the nutrients required to maintain it for life.

WIT is a simple, effective modality that should be as acceptable as oral hygiene is in the minds of people today. WIT addresses the cause of toxic overload in the abnormal colon flora. If the WIT procedure is followed from beginning to end, cleansing to maintenance, and if patient compliance is good, lasting results will be achieved in most cases.

WIT can be applied as a post-antibiotic therapy or as a pre-operative cleansing precaution. WIT is cost-effective, provides simple preventive care, and addresses current concerns about rising health care costs.

The sure mechanism for minimizing health care costs is to achieve maximum health by offering true prevention, which includes education. We all must make a choice whether to be satisfied with moderate health until something goes wrong or whether to take action to improve our health by strengthening our foundation. By applying the knowledge detailed in this book, the quality of health for all people will be increased, both in the present and in the future.

Knowing the true nature and function of the lactobacteria empowers people to play a fuller role and take increased responsibility for the well-being of themselves, their families, and friends. The purpose of this book is to educate by presenting facts. It is my hope that the information presented, along with the actual demonstration of the work, will stimulate further scientific research and development in this most needed field of the healing arts.

Ultimately, it is my hope that this procedure will be standardized and performed by well-trained, licensed practitioners throughout the world. The choice is ours to do nothing or do something, now that we know what we must do for our survival into the future. It is time to apply science. We are losing time.

The benefits of achieving a normal colon flora by utilizing WIT have been experienced by physicians, chiropractors, acupuncturists, homeopaths, naturopaths, and their patients. Health professionals accomplish better results with their clients once the colon soil has been addressed using WIT. The process of regaining health is a fascinating journey of discovery. Now the foundation of health has been laid on solid ground, the journey has just begun.

Will you be one more who achieves maximum health?

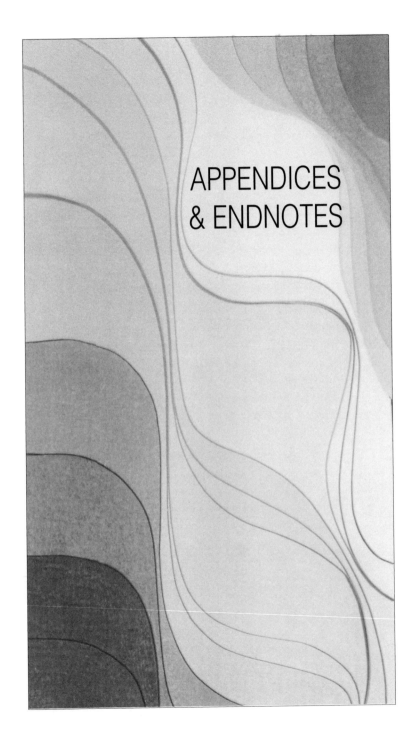
APPENDICES
& ENDNOTES

APPENDIX A

Resources

**American Association of Acupuncture
and Oriental Medicine (AAAOM)**
433 Front Street
Catasauqua, PA 18032-2506
Phone (610) 433-2448
Fax (610) 433-1832

Call or write for a referral to a licensed acupuncturist in your area. Most, but not all, are trained in Chinese herbal medicine.

Candida & Dysbiosis Information Foundation
(formerly Candida Research & Information Foundation)
P.O. Drawer F
College Station, TX 77841-5146
Phone (409) 694-8687

A private, non-profit health organization created for the purposes of public education and patient support services and for data collection on chronic illnesses suspected of having a fungal/mycotoxin etiology. A special emphasis is given to conditions characterized by an imbalanced intestinal microflora ecology. A referral list of MDs and other health care professionals who deal with these syndromes is available. Call or write for more information.

The Centers for Disease Control
Phone (404) 332-4555

Consumer information.

Jaffe Brothers
P.O. Box 636
Valley Center, CA 92082
Phone (619) 749-1133
Fax (619) 749-1282

National direct-mail source of top-quality organic grains. It offers organic nuts, seeds, virgin olive oil, and more. All are kept in a refrigerated warehouse and shipped via UPS. Jaffe Brothers have been in business for over 47 years. Call, write, or fax for a catalogue.

La Leche League International
1400 N. Meacham Road
P.O. Box 4079
Schaumburg, IL 60168-4079
Phone (800) 525-3243

The La Leche League, established in 1956, is a nationwide organization that offers practical and reliable information on breastfeeding.

MULTI-PURE™ Drinking Water System
Multi-Pure Corporation
P.O. Box 4179
Chatsworth, CA 91313-4179
Phone (800) 622-9206
Give them ID number 105185

Multi-Pure offers several water filter systems that have been independently certified by the National Sanitation Foundation. The Multi-Pure Drinking Water System removes lead, asbestos, many pesticides, *Cryptosporidium*, *Giardia* cysts, and chlorine from drinking water.

National Sanitation Foundation (NSF)
P.O. Box 130140
Ann Arbor, MI 48113-0140
Phone (313) 769-8010
Fax (313) 769-0109

An independent, not-for-profit organization of scientists, engineers, educators, and analysts. As a neutral agency, NSF has served in the areas of public health and the environment since 1944. One of its services is to evaluate, test, and inspect drinking water treatment systems. It certifies products that meet NSF standards and conducts unannounced audits at the manufacturing plants of these devices to ensure maintenance of NSF standards. For a complete listing of NSF certified water filter systems, request the booklet, *NSF Listings – Drinking Water Treatment Units.*

Price-Pottenger Nutrition Foundation
2667 Camino del Rio South, suite 109
San Diego, CA 92108
Phone (619) 574-7763
Fax (619) 574-1314

This non-profit organization is dedicated to promoting health and improving the environment. Its goal is to make optimum health available to everyone through education. The Price-Pottenger Nutrition Foundation library houses over 10,000 health-related books and remains one of the most trusted research collections nationwide. It offers a network and referral source for nutrition-oriented physicians.

World Research Foundation
15300 Ventura Boulevard #405
Sherman Oaks, CA 91403
Phone (818) 907-5483
Fax (818) 907-6044

This non-profit organization offers a unique, international information network. It will locate and disseminate information from around the world, encompassing both ancient and current data from traditional and non-traditional medicine. *World Research News* is its publication. Health information packets and books are available through WRF. It maintains offices in the United States, Europe, and the Far East. Excellent resource for both laypeople and health professionals.

WIT Program Recommended Products

I have used the following products extensively over the years with consistent, excellent results. There is no effective substitute for these outstanding products.

-David Webster

PRO FLORA™ 100% Natural Whey

Superior quality, sweet whey that is delicious, light, and fluffy. Classified as "edible whey" by the U.S. Department of Agriculture (U.S.D.A.), meaning it is made especially for human consumption. Mixes instantly in hot or cold water. This is the natural whey to feed and maintain your beneficial colon lactobacteria flora.

Kyo-Dophilus®

Highest-quality lactobacteria product on the market that I have found. Human source, high-count lactobacteria culture necessary for successful colonization and lasting results when used according to WIT. Heat stable, never needs refrigeration.

Kyolic®

Organically grown, odorless, aged liquid garlic extract. There are more than 150 published papers on the health benefits of Kyolic®, the original garlic extract. I recommend the liquid extract in the two-ounce, red-label bottle.

Genuine N-Zimes™

Plant enzymes that assist digestion of fat, starch, protein, and cellulose. Developed by enzyme researcher Dr. Edward Howell.

WIT KIT© Self-Help Enema System

Four simple steps to help you achieve colon health. Contains all the products listed above, with an enema kit and other items necessary to perform Webster Implant Technique© at home. Includes complete instructions with questions and answers.

Since I first published my booklet *Acidophilus & Colon Health* in 1980, I have received requests from people all over the country who wanted to experience WIT. Because of these requests, and since no one other than myself is currently trained to administer WIT, I decided to offer WIT in the form of a self-help kit. WIT KIT© was designed to offer an effective, safe, preventive method to achieve colon health.

WIT KIT© is not meant to take the place of proper medical care. WIT KIT© does not treat or cure any condition. Always consult your health care provider for any condition or illness.

WIT KIT© can be used

• after a course of antibiotics to restore the beneficial colon flora

• after *Candida* or parasites have been eradicated, to restore normal colon flora and to prevent relapse

• after traveling to Third World countries as a preventive measure

• as a preventive measure to provide a foundation for good health and immunity

For brochure and information:
ADVANCED HEALTH SOLUTIONS
PO Box 937
Cardiff, California 92007
Phone (800) 943-0054

Joanne
760-721-4759
cell
760-500-5494

Kyo-Green®

Chlorophyll is nature's disinfectant in the bloodstream. Kyo-Green® combines barley grass, wheat grass, kelp, chlorella, and brown rice. This superior product is a strong immune enhancer. It has a superb taste and mixes instantly.

APPENDIX C

Recommended Reading

Life, Death and the Immune System. *Scientific American*, 1993.

Dunne LJ. *Nutrition Almanac.* McGraw-Hill Publishing Company, New York, 1990.

Erasmus U. *Fats that Heal, Fats that Kill.* Alive Books, Burnaby, BC Canada, 1993.

Erdmann R, Jones M. *Fats that can save your life: The Critical Role of Fats and Oils in Health and Disease.* Progressive Health Publishing, Encinitas, CA. 1995.

Gittleman AL. *Guess What Came to Dinner: Parasites and Your Health.* Avery Publishing Group, Inc., Wayne, NJ, 1993.

Howell E. *Enzyme Nutrition: The Food Enzyme Concept.* Avery Publishing Group, Inc., Wayne, NJ, 1985.

Lau B. *Garlic for Health.* Lotus Light Publications, Wilmot, WI, 1988.

Levy SB. *The Antibiotic Paradox: How Miracle Drugs Are Destroying the Miracle.* Plenum Press, New York, 1992.

Long JW. *The Essential Guide to Prescription Drugs.* HarperPerennial, New York, 1995.

Pitchford P. *Healing with Whole Foods: Oriental Traditions and Modern Nutrition.* North Atlantic Books, Berkeley, CA,1993.

Rombauer IS, Becker MR. *Joy of Cooking.* The Bobbs-Merrill Company, Inc., New York, 1975.

Webster D. *Acidophilus & Colon Health.* Hygeia Publishing, Cardiff, CA,1995.

Endnotes

Preface: An Unexpected Avenue: The Toxic Colon

1. Thomas CL. *Taber's Cyclopedic Medical Dictionary*. 17th edition. FA Davis Company, Philadelphia, 1993.

Chapter 1   In the Beginning

1. Donaldson RM. Normal Bacterial Populations of the Intestine and Their Relation to Intestinal Function. *The New England Journal of Medicine*. 1964;270(18):941.
2. Haenel H. Human Normal and Abnormal Gastrointestinal Flora. *The American Journal of Clinical Nutrition*. 1970;23(11):1433.
3. Ibid:1433.
4. Brock TD, Madigan MT. *Biology of Microorganisms*. Sixth edition. Prentice Hall, Englewood Cliffs, NJ, 1991:393.
5. Jawetz E, Melnick JL, Adelberg EA. *Review of Medical Microbiology*. 16th edition. Lange Medical Publications, Los Altos, CA, 1984:293.
6. Lappe M. *When Antibiotics FAIL: Restoring the Ecology of the Body*. North Atlantic Books, Berkeley, CA, 1986:50-51.
7. Hamilton E. The Lost Art of Breast-Feeding. *Women's Times*. San Diego, CA, September 1993:33-34.
8. Wilson NW, Hamburger RN. Allergy to cow's milk in the first year of life and its prevention. *Annals of Allergy*. November 1988;61(5):323-327.
9. Hamilton E. op. cit.
10. Sassen ML, et al. Breast Feeding and Acute Otitis Media. *American Journal of Otolaryngology*. September-October 1994;15(5):351-357.

Chapter 2   The Protective Shield: Immunity And The Colon

1. Joklik WK, Willett HP. *Zinsser Microbiology.* 16th edition. Appleton-Century-Crofts, New York, 1976:409.

2. Burtis G, Davis J, Martin S. *Applied Nutrition and Diet Therapy.* WB Saunders Company, Philadelphia, 1988:45.

3. Seeley RR, Stephens TD, Tate P. *Anatomy and Physiology.* Times Mirror/Mosby College Publishing, St. Louis, MO, 1989.

4. Miller MA, Drakontides AB, Leavell LC. *Kimber-Gray-Stackpole's Anatomy and Physiology.* Seventeenth edition. Macmillan Publishing Co, Inc, New York, 1977.

5. Thomas CL. *Taber's Cyclopedic Medical Dictionary.* 17th edition. FA Davis Company, Philadelphia, 1993.

6. Spiro HM. *Clinical Gastroenterology.* Fourth edition. McGraw-Hill, Inc., New York, 1993:526.

7. Pelczar MJJ, Reid RD. *Microbiology.* Second edition. McGraw-Hill Book Company, New York, 1965:26.

8. Snyder RG, Traeger CH, Fineman S, Zoll CA. Colonic Stasis in Chronic Arthritis. *Archives of Physical Therapy, X-Ray, Radium.* October 1939;14:610-617.

9. Hibben JS. Irrigation of the Colon. *Archives of Physical Therapy.* 1940;21:33-40.

10. Traut EF. The Gastrointestinal Tract in Chronic Rheumatism. *Archives of Physical Therapy.* 1934;15:479-482.

11. Fishbaugh EC. Colon Disease and Its Therapy in Relation to Chronic Arthritis. *Archives of Physical Therapy.* July 1939;20:411-416.

12. Gibson GR, Roberfroid MB. Dietary Modulation of the Human Colonic Microbiota: Introducing the Concept of Prebiotics. *Journal of Nutrition.* 1995;125:1401-1412.

13. Thomas CL. *Taber's Cyclopedic Medical Dictionary.* 13th edition. FA Davis Company, Philadelphia, 1977.

14. Sneath PHA, Mair NS, Sharpe ME, Holt JG. *Bergey's Manual® of Systematic Bacteriology.* Volume 2. Williams & Wilkins, Baltimore, MD, 1986.

15. Holt JG, Krieg NR, Sneath PHA, Staley JT, Williams ST. *Bergey's Manual® of Determinative Bacteriology.* Ninth edition. Williams

& Wilkins, Baltimore, MD, 1994.

16. Sneath PHA, Mair NS, Sharpe ME, Holt JG. *Bergey's Manual® of Systematic Bacteriology.* Volume 2. Williams & Wilkins, Baltimore, MD, 1986.

17. Joklik WK, Willett HP. *Zinsser Microbiology.* 16th edition. Appleton-Century-Crofts, New York, 1976.

18. Mackowiak PA. The Normal Microbial Flora. *The New England Journal of Medicine.* July 8, 1982;307(2):88.

Chapter 3 A Crisis In Health Care: The Neglected Colon

1. Erasmus U. *Fats that Heal, Fats that Kill.* Second edition. Alive Books, Burnaby BC, Canada, 1993.

Chapter 4 The War: The Visible Army Versus the Invisible Army

1. Levy SB. *The Antibiotic Paradox: How Miracle Drugs Are Destroying the Miracle.* Plenum Press, New York, 1992.

2. Adler J. The Age Before Miracles. *Newsweek.* March 28, 1994:52.

3. Begley S. The End of Antibiotics. *Newsweek.* 1994:47-52.

4. Cowley G. Too Much of a Good Thing. *Newsweek.* March 28, 1994:50-51.

5. Lappe M. *When Antibiotics FAIL: Restoring the Ecology of the Body.* North Atlantic Books, Berkeley, CA, 1986.

Chapter 5 Antibiotics: Defense Betrayed

1. Pelczar MJJ, Reid RD. *Microbiology.* Second edition. McGraw-Hill Book Company, New York, 1965:331.

2. Ibid:331.

3. Ibid:331.

4. Levy SB. *The Antibiotic Paradox: How Miracle Drugs Are Destroying the Miracle.* Plenum Press, New York, 1992:50.

5. Ibid:114.

6. Press Release. "Silver" Tooth Fillings are Implicated in the Spread of Antibiotic Resistant Bacteria - an Increasing Problem in Medi-

cine Today. The University of Calgary, Calgary, Alberta, Canada, April 1, 1993.

7. Levy SB. op cit:84.
8. Ibid:145-147.
9. *A guide to the use of diagnostic instruments in Eye, Ear, Nose and Throat examinations.* Welch Allyn, 1991.
10. Lappe M. *When Antibiotics FAIL: Restoring the Ecology of the Body.* North Atlantic Books, Berkeley, CA 1986:196.

Chapter 6 Candida

1. Young G, Krasner RI, Yudkofsky PL. Interactions of Oral Strains of *Candida Albicans* and Lactobacilli. *Journal of Bacteriology.* 1956; 72(4):528.
2. Wyngaarden JB, Smith JLH, Bennett JC. *Cecil Textbook of Medicine.* 19th edition. WB Saunders Company, Philadelphia, PA, 1988:1898-1901.
3. Ibid:1898-1901.
4. Ibid:1898-1901.
5. Ibid:1898-1899.
6. Ibid:1898-1901.
7. Dismukes WE, Wade JS, Lee JY, Dockery BK, Hain JD. A Randomized, Double-Blind Trial of Nystatin Therapy for the Candidiasis Hypersensitivity Syndrome. *The New England Journal of Medicine.* December 20, 1990;323(25):1717-1723.
8. Wyngaarden JB, Smith JLH, Bennett JC. op cit:1900.
9. Young G, Krasner RI, Yudkofsky PL. op cit:525.
10. Joklik WK, Willett HP. *Zinsser Microbiology.* 16th edition. Appleton-Century-Crofts, New York, 1976.
11. Young G, Krasner RI, Yudkofsky PL. op cit:525.

Chapter 7 Parasites: Opportunistic Organisms

1. Markell EK, Voge M, John DT. *Medical Parasitology.* 7th edition. W.B. Saunders Company, Philadelphia, 1992:14-15.
2. Ibid:263.

3. Katz M, Despommier DD, Gwadz RW. *Parasitic Diseases*. 2nd edition. Springer-Verlag, New York, 1989:11.

4. Muller R, Baker JR. *Medical Paristology*. J.B. Lippincott Company, Philadelphia, 1990:97.

5. Ibid:97.

6. Ibid:97.

7. Markell EK, Voge M, John DT. op cit:264.

8. Ibid:285.

9. Ibid:226-260.

10. Ibid:14,63,75.

11. Ibid:63-69.

12. Ibid:63-69.

13. Ibid:14-15.

14. Ibid.

Chapter 8 Bacterial Polluters

1. Fatalities Attributed to Entering Manure Waste Pits - Minnesota, 1992. *Morbidity and Mortality Weekly Report*. May 7, 1993;42(17):325-329.

2. Immerman A. Evidence for Intestinal Toxemia: An Inescapable Clinical Phenomenon. *The American Chiropractic Association Journal of Chiropractic*. April 1979;13,S-25:1-19.

3. Baron EJ, Finegold SM. *Bailey & Scott's Diagnostic Microbiology*. Eighth edition. The C.V. Mosby Company, Princeton, NJ, 1990:363.

4. Ibid:368.

5. Ibid:367.

6. The Centers for Disease Control information line recording. December 1994.

7. Brock TD, Madigan MT. *Biology of Microorganisms*. Sixth edition. Prentice Hall, Englewood Cliffs, NJ, 1991:395.

8. Finegold SM, Attebery HR, Sutter VL. Effect of diet on human fecal flora: comparison of Japanese and American diets. *The American Journal of Clinical Nutrition*. December 1974;27:1456-1469.

9. Miller BA, Ries LAG, Hankey BF, et al. *SEER Cancer Statistics Re-*

view: 1973-1990. NIH Pub. No. 93-2789 National Cancer Institute; Bethesda, MD, 1993.

10. Drasar S, Hill MJ. Intestinal bacteria and cancer. *The American Journal of Clinical Nutrition.* December 1972;25:1399-1404.

11. Ibid.

12. Newmark HL, Lupton JR. Determinants and Consequences of Colonic Luminal pH: Implications for Colon Cancer. *Nutrition and Cancer.* 1990;14(3-4):161-173.

13. Malhotra SL. Faecal urobilinogen levels and pH of stools in population groups with different incidence of cancer of the colon, and their possible role in aetiology. *Journal of the Royal Society of Medicine.* September 1982;75.

14. Hill MJ, Goddard P, Williams REO. Gut Bacteria and Aetiology of Cancer of the Breast. *The Lancet.* August 28, 1971:472-473.

15. Drasar S, Hill MJ. op cit.

16. Hill MJ, Goddard P, Williams REO. op cit.

17. Drasar S, Hill MJ. op cit.

18. Javitt NB, Budai K, Miller DG, Cahan AC, Raju U, Levitz M. Breast-gut connection: origin of chenodeoxycholic acid in breast cyst fluid. *The Lancet.* March 12, 1994;343:633-634.

19. Finegold SM, Attebery HR, Sutter VL. op cit.

20. Gorbach SL. Estrogens, Breast Cancer, and Intestinal Flora. *Reviews of Infectious Diseases.* March - April 1984;6,Supplement 1.

21. Drasar S, Hill MJ. op cit.

22. Finegold SM, Attebery HR, Sutter VL. op cit.

23. Hill MJ, Goddard P, Williams REO. op cit.

24. Drasar S, Hill MJ. op cit.

25. Javitt NB, Budai K, Miller DG, Cahan AC, Raju U, Levitz M. op cit.

26. Finegold SM, Attebery HR, Sutter VL. op cit.

27. Hill MJ, Goddard P, Williams REO. op cit.

28. Lee JR. *Natural Progesterone: The Multiple roles of a Remarkable Hormone.* BLL Publishing, Sepastopol, CA, 1993.

29. Aries VC, Crowther JS, Drasar BS, Hill MJ, Ellis FR. The Effect of a Strict Vegetarian Diet on the Faecal Flora and Faecal Steroid Concentration. *Journal of Pathology.* 1971;103:54-56.

30. Javitt NB, Budai K, Miller DG, Cahan AC, Raju U, Levitz M. op cit.

31. Hill MJ, Goddard P, Williams REO. op cit.

32. Drasar S, Hill MJ. op cit.

33. Cummings JH, Hill MJ, Jenkins DJA, Pearson JR, Wiggins HS. Changes in fecal composition and colonic function due to cereal fiber. *American Journal of Clinical Nutrition.* 1976;29:1468-1473.

34. Finegold SM, Attebery HR, Sutter VL. op cit.

35. Donaldson RM. Normal Bacterial Populations of the Intestine and their Relation to Intestinal Function. *The New England Journal of Medicine.* 1964;270(18):938-945.

36. Maier BR, Flynn MA, Burton GC, Tsutakawa RK, Hentges DJ. Effects of a high-beef diet on bowel flora: a preliminary report. *American Journal of Clinical Nutrition.* 1974;27:1456-1469.

37. Cummings JH, Hill MJ, Jenkins DJA, Pearson JR, Wiggins HS. Changes in fecal composition and colonic function due to cereal fiber. *American Journal of Clinical Nutrition.* 1976;29:1468-1473.

38. Finegold SM, Attebery HR, Sutter VL. op cit.

39. Walker ARP, Walker BF, Walker AJ. Faecal pH, dietary fibre intake, and proneness to colon cancer in four South African populations. *British Journal of Cancer.* 1986;53:489-495.

Chapter 9 Autointoxication Explained

1. Brown L, editor. *The New Shorter Oxford English Dictionary.* Thumb Index Edition. Clarendon Press, Oxford, England, 1993.

2. Thomas CL. *Taber's Cyclopedic Medical Dictionary.* 17th edition. FA Davis Company, Philadelphia, 1993.

3. Ibid.

4. Empringham J. *Intestinal Gardening for the Prolongation of Youth.* Revised and Reprinted with New Chapters. Health Education Society, Los Angeles, CA, 1941:18-19.

5. Spiro HM. *Clinical Gastroenterology.* Fourth edition. McGraw-Hill, Inc., New York, 1993:415.

6. Miller MA, Drakontides AB, Leavell LC. *Kimber-Gray-Stackpole's Anatomy and Physiology.* Seventeenth edition. Macmillan Publishing Co., Inc., New York, 1977.

7. Thomas CL. op cit.
8. Seeley RR, Stephens TD, Tate P. *Anatomy and Physiology*. Times Mirror/Mosby College Publishing, St. Louis, MO, 1989.
9. Rhoades R, Pflanzer R. *Human Physiology*. Second edition. Saunders College Publishing, Philadelphia, 1992.
10. Barral J-P. *Visceral Manipulation II*. Eastland Press, Seattle, WA, 1989:99.
11. Seeley RR, Stephens TD, Tate P. op cit:635.
12. Bland JS. A Functional Approach to Mental Illness - A New Paradigm for Managing Brain Biochemical Disturbances. *Townsend Letter for Doctors,* Reprinted with permission from *The Journal of Orthomolecular Medicine*. December 1994:1336.
13. Empringham J. *Gland Reactivation and the New Knowledge of the Body*. Health Education Society, Los Angeles, CA 1940:161.
14. Ibid:145.

Chapter 10   Aging and Mental Health: The Colon Connection

1. Empringham J. *Invisible Friends of the Body*. Health Education Society, Los Angeles, CA, 1944:301-303.
2. Empringham J. *Intestinal Gardening for the Prolongation of Youth*. Revised and reprinted with new chapters. Health Education Society, Los Angeles, CA, 1941:11-17.
3. Mitsuoka T. Intestinal Flora and Aging. *Nutrition Reviews*. December 1992;50:438-446.
4. Kaiser NW. Colonic Therapy in Mental Disease. *The Ohio State Medical Journal*. June 1930;26:510.
5. Ibid.
6. Ibid:511
7. Ibid.
8. Ibid:512.
9. Ibid.
10. Bland JS. A Functional Approach to Mental Illness - A New Paradigm for Managing Brain Biochemical Disturbances. *Townsend Letter for Doctors,* Reprinted with permission from *The Journal of Orthomolecular Medicine*. December 1994:1335-1341.

11. Ibid:1336.
12. Ibid:1338.

Chapter 11   Colon in the Quest for Health

1. Friedenwald J, Morrison S. The History of the Enema with Some Notes on Related Procedures (Part I). *Bulletin of History of Medicine.* 1940;8:68-114.
2. Knox JG. Letter: Colonics & Enemas. *Townsend Letter for Doctors.* February/March 1994:216-219.
3. Friedenwald J, Morrison S. op cit (Part I):77-79.
4. Friedenwald J, Morrison S. op cit (Part I).
5. Friedenwald J, Morrison S. op cit (Part I):74.
6. Friedenwald J, Morrison S. The History of the Enema with Some Notes on Related Procedures (Part II). *Bulletin of History of Medicine.* 1940;8:239-276.
7. Friedenwald J, Morrison S. op cit (Part II):261.
8. Friedenwald J, Morrison S. op cit (Part I):77.
9. Friedenwald J, Morrison S. op cit (Part I):91.
10. Friedenwald J, Morrison S. op cit (Part I):91.
11. Friedenwald J, Morrison S. op cit (Part I):94.
12. Friedenwald J, Morrison S. op cit (Part II):244.
13. Friedenwald J, Morrison S. op cit (Part II):245.
14. Friedenwald J, Morrison S. op cit (Part II):258.

Chapter 12   The Fathers of Colon Microbiology

1. Empringham J. *Invisible Friends of the Body.* Health Education Society, Los Angeles, CA, 1944:9.
2. James W. *Immunization: The Reality Behind the Myth.* Bergin & Garvey, Westport, CT, 1988.
3. Ibid.
4. *Nobel Lectures including Presentation Speeches and Laureates' Biographies: 1922-1941.* Published for the Nobel Foundation by Elsevier Publishing Company, Amsterdam-London-New York, 1965.
5. Empringham J. op cit:14-15.

6. Thomas CL. *Taber's Cyclopedic Medical Dictionary*. 17th edition. FA Davis Company, Philadelphia, 1993.
7. Empringham J. op cit:30.

Chapter 13   Microbiology and Colon Hygiene: A Good Marriage

1. Barghoorn ES. Colonic Therapy: Its Relation to Medical Practice. *The American Journal of Physical Therapy*. February, 1932;8:304-306.
2. Hughens HV. A Bio-Physiotherapeutic Procedure in the Treatment of Non-Malignant Diseases of the Colon. *United States Naval Medical Bulletin*. May 1925;XXII(5):511.
3. Ibid:526.

Chapter 14   A Giant Step Backward

1. Brock TD, Madigan MT. *Biology of Microorganisms*. Sixth edition. Prentice Hall, Englewood Cliffs, NJ, 1991:392-394.
2. Stoy D, et.al. Cholesterol-Lowering Effects of Ready-To-Eat Cereal Containing Psyllium. *Journal of the American Dietetic Association*. 1993;93(8):910-911.
3. Damrau F, The Value of Bentonite for Diarrhea. *Medical Annals of the District of Columbia*. June 1961;30(6).

Chapter 15   Setting the Record Straight: The Definitive Report on Lactobacteria

1. *Mosby's Medical & Nursing Dictionary*. 2nd edition. The C.V. Mosby Company, Princeton, NJ, 1986.
2. Sneath PHA, Mair NS, Sharpe ME, Holt JG. *Bergey's Manual® of Systematic Bacteriology*. Volume 2. Williams & Wilkins, Baltimore, MD, 1986:1217.
3. Ibid:1212.
4. Sneath PHA, Mair NS, Sharpe ME, Holt JG. op cit.
5. Holt JG, Krieg NR, Sneath PHA, Staley JT, Williams ST. *Bergey's Manual® of Determinative Bacteriology*. Ninth edition. Williams & Wilkins, Baltimore, MD, 1994.

6. Kovac Laboratories, Inc. product information sheet. Oceanside, CA, circa 1983.
7. Webster D. *Intestinal Gardening: excerpts of Dr. James Empringham.* M.C. Winchester Publisher, Hermosa Beach, CA, 1986:21.
8 Mackowiak PA. The Normal Microbial Flora. *The New England Journal of Medicine.* July 8, 1982;307(2):88.
9. Ibid.
10. Goldin BR, Gorbach SL. The effect of milk and lactobacillus feeding on human intestinal bacterial enzyme activity. *The American Journal of Clinical Nutrition.* May 1984;39:756-761.
11. Ibid.
12. Wyngaarden JB, Smith JLH, Bennett JC. *Cecil Textbook of Medicine.* 19th edition. WB Saunders Company, Philadelphia, 1988:1658.
13. Brock TD, Madigan MT. *Biology of Microorganisms.* Sixth edition. Prentice Hall, Englewood Cliffs, NJ, 1991:392.
14. Wyngaarden JB, Smith JLH, Bennett JC. op cit.
15. Mackowiak PA. op cit.

Chapter 16   *Webster Implant Technique: Colon Hygiene into the 21st Century*

1. Robins-Browne RM, Levine MM. The fate of ingested lactobacilli in the proximal small intestine. *The American Journal of Clinical Nutrition.* April 1981;34:514-519.
2. Hughes VL, Hillier SL. Microbiologic Characteristics of Lactobacillus Products Used for Colonization of the Vagina. *Obstetrics & Gynecology.* February 1990;75(2):244-248.
3. Mackowiak PA. The Normal Microbial Flora. *The New England Journal of Medicine.* July 8, 1982;307(2):84.
4. Ibid:88.
5. Ibid:84.
6. Davis JG. The Microbiology of Yoghourt. In: Carr JG, Cutting CV, Whiting GC, editors. *Fourth Long Ashton Symposium.* Long Ashton Research Station, University of Bristol, Academic Press: September 1973:19-21.

Chapter 17   Whey of Life

1. Young G, Krasner RI, Yudkofsky PL. Interactions of Oral Strains of *Candida Albicans* and *Lactobacilli. Journal of Bacteriology.* 1956; 72(4):526.

2. *Handbook of Nonprescription Drugs.* 10th edition. American Pharmaceutical Association, Washington, DC,1993.

3. Thomas CL. *Taber's Cyclopedic Medical Dictionary.* 17th edition. FA Davis Company, Philadelphia, 1993.

4. Ibid.

5. Leibovitz B. Whey Protein: A Unique Source of Protein. *Muscular Development Magazine;* 1989.

6. *The New Grolier Multimedia Encyclopedia.* Macintosh Version, Release 6. Grolier, Inc, Danbury, CT, 1993.

7. Friedenwald J, Morrison S. The History of the Enema with some Notes on Related Procedures (Part II). *Bulletin of History of Medicine.* 1940;8:239-276.

8. National Academy of Sciences. *Improvement of Protein Nutriture.* Committee on Amino Acids, Food and Nutrition Board, National Research Council, Washington, DC, 1974.

9. Leibovitz B. op cit.

10. Brody T. *Nutritional Biochemistry.* Academic Press, San Diego, CA, 1994.

11. Austin PR, Brine CJ, Castle JE, Zikakis JP. Chitin: New facets of research. *Science.* May 15, 1981;212(4496):749-753.

12. Bond JHJ, Levitt MD. Fate of Soluble Carbohydrate in the Colon of Rats and Man. *The Journal of Clinical Investigation.* May 1976;57:1158-1164.

13. Burtis G, Davis J, Martin S. *Applied Nutrition and Diet Therapy.* WB Saunders Company, Philadelphia, 1988.

14. Mitsuoka T, Hidaka H, Eida T. Effect of fructo-oligosaccharides on intestinal microflora. *Die Nahrung.* 1987;31(5-6):427-436.

15. *Handbook of Nonprescription Drugs.* op cit.

16. Morris GB, Porter RL, Meyer KF. The Bacteriologic Analysis of the Fecal Flora of Children with notes on the changes produced by a carbohydrate diet. *The Journal of Infectious Diseases.* 1919;25:376.

Chapter 18 Golden Grains

1. Thomas CL. *Taber's Cyclopedic Medical Dictionary.* 17th edition.
    FA Davis Company, Philadelphia, 1993.
2. Ibid.
3. Blaine JTR. *Mental Health Through Nutrition.* The Citadel Press,
    New York, 1969:19-22.
4. Cheraskin E, Ringsdorf Jr WM. *Psychodietetics: Food as the Key to
    Emotional Health.* Stein and Day Publishers, New York, 1974:82-83.

Chapter 19 Fasting and Other Food Follies

1. Hill MJ, Goddard P, Williams REO. Gut Bacteria and Aetiology of
    Cancer of the Breast. *The Lancet.* August 28, 1971:472-473.
2. Drasar S, Hill MJ. Intestinal bacteria and cancer. *The American
    Journal of Clinical Nutrition.* December 1972;25:1399-1404.
3. Cummings JH, Hill MJ, Jenkins DJA, Pearson JR, Wiggins HS.
    Changes in fecal composition and colonic function due to cereal
    fiber. *American Journal of Clinical Nutrition.* 1976;29:1468-1473.
4. Finegold SM, Attebery HR, Sutter VL. Effect of diet on human
    fecal flora: comparison of Japanese and American diets. *The
    American Journal of Clinical Nutrition.* December 1974;27:1456-
    1469.
5. Erasmus U. *Fats that Heal, Fats that Kill.* Second edition. Alive
    Books, Burnaby BC, Canada, 1993.
6. Budwig DJ. *Flax Oil as a True Aid against Arthritis, Heart Infarc-
    tion, Cancer and other Diseases.* Apple Publishing Company,
    Vancouver, BC, Canada, 1992.
7. Erdmann R, Jones M. *Fats that can save your life: the Critical Role of
    Fats and Oils in Health and Disease..* Progressive Health Publish-
    ing, Encinitas, CA. 1995.
8. Bland JS. A Functional Approach to Mental Illness - A New Para-
    digm for Managing Brain Biochemical Disturbances. *Townsend
    Letter for Doctors,* Reprinted with permission from *The Journal of
    Orthomolecular Medicine.* December 1994:1336.
9. Leviton R. Profile: Leon Chaitow. *East West.* September/October
    1991;21(8):44-46.

10. Bland JS. op cit.

11. Leviton R. op cit:44-46.

12. Bland JS. op cit.

13. Yanick P. Functional Correlates of pH in Accelerated Molecular and Tissue Aging, *Townsend Letter for Doctors*, May 1995:34-38.

14. Press Release. "Silver" Tooth fillings are Implicated in the Spread of Antibiotic Resistant Bacteria - An Increasing Problem in Medicine Today. The University of Calgary, Calgary, Alberta, Canada, April 1, 1993.

Chapter 20 Nutrition, Lifestyle, and Colon Health

1. EPA Finds High Lead Levels Across Nation. *Nutrition Week*; May 21, 1993.

2. Marchesani RB. *Cryptosporidium* Outbreak Hits Milwaukee; Seven Deaths Linked to Contaminated Water. *Infectious Disease News.* May 1993;6(5):1.

3. Howell E. *Enzyme Nutrition: The Food Enzyme Concept.* Avery Publishing Group, Inc, Wayne, NJ, 1985.

4. Gerber R. *Vibrational Medicine: New Choices for Healing Ourselves.* Bear & Company, Santa Fe, NM, 1988:64.

5. Brown BB. *New Mind, New Body.* Bantam Books, New York, 1974:353.

6. *The New Grolier Multimedia Encyclopedia.* Macintosh Version, Release 6. Grolier, Inc., Danbury, CT, 1993.

Chapter 21 Achieve Maximum Health

1. Begley S. The End of Antibiotics. *Newsweek.* 1994:47-52.

2. Levy SB. *The Antibiotic Paradox: How Miracle Drugs Are Destroying the Miracle.* Plenum Press, New York, 1992.

Index

C

E

O

P

U

V

W

About the Author

David Webster is a health research author and colon hygienist. His area of specialty is colon health, which he has researched for 20 years, compiling 100 years of data from America, Europe, and Japan. He authored *Acidophilus & Colon Health*, now in its sixth edition, a best-selling booklet in health food stores since 1980. David has been a guest speaker on several radio talk shows, has instructed at a local college, and gives frequent lectures.

David is the originator of Webster Implant Technique (WIT), an effective method of colon hygiene that is based on his research. He has six years of clinical experience with WIT, which reestablishes the normal colon pH and flora. WIT offers a unique approach to health, combining microbiological facts with principles of colon health.

David's new book, *Achieve Maximum Health*, is a definitive report that reveals the important role of the colon flora in immune function and health. David Webster is here to set the record straight in the area of colon health, separating the many popular myths from the scientific facts.

Notes